Breathwork

How a Daily Breathing Practice Can Drastically Improve Your Mind, Body, and Spirit

By Jane Rivers

Contents

Introduction

When it comes to humans, animals, and just about every single living thing that you can think of, they are going to have one thing in common: breathing. This is why the absolute first concern an emergency responder will look for in any type of emergency will be if the distressed person is breathing. This is an essential question as it will also be the first one asked about newborn babies, and the last one asked when somebody is dying. With all of this being said, have you ever wondered why breathing is so important? And since breathing is so vital, are you then able to practice and improve how you breathe through breathwork, with the ultimate goal of improving your mind, body, and spirit?

These are all excellent questions, and we will get to them momentarily. In order to understand how to improve your body, mind, and spirit using breathwork, you will need to know how breathing works within your body. Once you fathom this process, you will be better equipped to harness the powers and benefits that it can bring you.

Now you may be thinking, "I already know how breathing works!" You don't need to do anything, as your body will do all of your breathing automatically, right? The answer is going to be yes, and this is technically true, that your body is going to be doing most of the work involved with breathing on its own without you needing to think about it. However, studies have proven that if you can understand and harness the power of your breathing using breathwork, the number of benefits you will receive will be tremendous! You will feel happier, healthier, and more aware, just to name a few.

But as mentioned earlier, we will get to that shortly. Until then, here is exactly how breathing happens in your body and how you can use breathwork to increase its benefits.

Chapter 1: Breathing and Your

Body

Before getting started with how breathing works in your body, let's first clarify exactly what 'breathwork' is. Breathwork is defined as any type of conscious breathing technique or exercise. Breathwork is commonly used to help improve your physical, spiritual, and mental well-being. When practicing breathwork, you will be intentionally changing your regular breathing pattern. The practice of breathwork has recently seen a massive surge in popularity. Many people will attest to the fact that it can help you fall into deep relaxation or even help you feel more energetic.

Now that you know what breathwork is, how can the simple act of breathing help you to increase your mind, body, and awareness?

Breathing 101

For your body to operate at maximal efficiency, it will require energy to help fuel everything that occurs. For example, every time your body contracts a muscle or maintains a resting state in your body's neurons, it is going to be using energy. The energy available in your body is not unlimited, which means that you are going to need to somehow obtain more of it to keep your body working. So how is this done, you are wondering?

Plants get their energy by taking sunlight and then turning it into carbohydrates (or sugars), which they then use to function in a process known as photosynthesis. Humans are not able to do this. While you use the energy found in carbohydrates to fuel the different reactions within your body, the process is much different from what it is in plants.

For the human body to produce the energy that it requires daily, it combines oxygen with sugar. This means that you will need to accumulate both oxygen and sugar, ultimately requiring your body to work to fill this need. In fact, most of the energy you do have will be used to acquire more sugar and oxygen so that you can produce even more energy.

You already know that the oxygen you need for this reaction will come from the air that you breathe, but where do the carbohydrates come from? The carbohydrates required to complete this entire process come from plants or animals that have eaten these same plants. When oxygen and sugars are combined within the human body, your body will have all of the components needed to produce more energy.

On a side note, if you are wondering why the world doesn't run out of oxygen since every person and animal needs it to survive, the answer is that the earth's plants supply it. You see, plants use the sunlight along with carbon dioxide in the air to create the energy they need. This same plant will then release oxygen as a byproduct. Conversely, humans and other animals will use this same oxygen that the plant has released along with carbohydrates to create the energy that they need to survive, releasing carbon dioxide as a waste product. As you can see, plants and animals are going to need each other to complete their cycle of energy production!

To sum it up, for your body to produce energy, you will need to use oxygen from the air that you breathe and combine it with sugars that you get from the carbohydrates that you eat.

Oxygen and Energy: How They Work in Your Body

For your body to gain the energy that it requires to operate at an optimal level, it will need to release the energy that is contained within the chemical bonds of the molecules that you consume, for example, sugars. When you eat foods (loaded with proteins and carbohydrates), they will then be digested in your gastrointestinal tract. Once these foods have been digested, they turn into smaller molecules (such as amino acids and sugars) that can pass into your bloodstream. In the bloodstream, these molecules are then transported to the cells of your body, where mitochondria will begin to break down their chemical bonds, freeing the energy that they contain. The cells of your body require oxygen to complete this process. Every one of the cells in your body requires energy to function properly, which means you will need a lot of oxygen.

Once the cells of your body breakdown the molecules and their energy is released, the energy will then be stored in a special chemical compound known as ATP, or adenosine triphosphate, which contains three phosphates. If your body needs more energy to carry out a function or activity, this stored ATP will be broken down, ultimately releasing its stored energy. Your body will then be able to use this energy to complete the function or activity that is at hand.

To sum this up, your body is going to require oxygen to break down the foods that you eat, ultimately turning that food into energy. Your body will then store that energy for a time when it needs it to perform a function or activity, allowing you to do so without any problems.

Your 2 Respirations: Internal and External

You probably know that your lungs supply all of the oxygen your body needs from the outside air, bringing that same air into your body, transporting it via blood and your cardiovascular system so you can obtain the energy that you require to function. As you breathe air in, oxygen will then enter your lungs and be diffused into your bloodstream. This is where it will be taken to your heart and pumped into all of the cells in your body. Simultaneously, carbon dioxide (the waste product from breaking down the sugars within the cells of your body) will then be diffused into your blood, taking the oxygen's spot. The carbon dioxide will then be diffused into your lungs, finally being expelled from your body every time that you breathe out.

When you breathe in, you take in oxygen that will then be diffused into the cells of your body for them to create energy. At the very same time, carbon dioxide will be exchanged for that oxygen, effectively eliminating the byproduct of the energy your body produced. This gas exchange happens within your lungs (which is known as external respiration), as well as in your body's cells, which is called internal respiration (or cellular respiration).

Getting Air into Your Lungs

When you breathe in to get air into your body, your respiratory system does all of the work. This system consists of a conduction zone, as well as a respiratory zone. The conduction zone is responsible for bringing in the air from your external environment and transporting it into your lungs through various air traveling tubes. These include:

- The naval cavity
- Your pharynx (which is the part of your throat that sits right behind your mouth and nasal cavity)
- Your voice box, or larynx
- The trachea, or windpipe
- Many different bronchi and bronchioles

While these all help your body get the air you breathe into your lungs, they are responsible for much more than just transporting air. These tubes also work together to:

- Warm up the incoming air
- Filter any tiny particles that may be in the air
- Increase the air's moisture content to ease the gas exchange process within your lungs

Your nasal cavity has many little capillaries that constantly bring warm blood to your cold nose. It is this warmth that will be diffused into the incoming cold air as it enters your nose. So essentially, the blood in your nose aids in warming the cold outside air that enters your body.

Once the air has entered your body, the lining of the larynx and pharynx (which form your upper respiratory tract), plus the lining in your trachea (also called your lower respiratory tract), work to clean the air you breathe. Both the upper and lower respiratory tract have cilia or little hairs on them. These hairs trap many of the smaller, airborne particles that may have entered your body with the air, such as dust. This process prevents these airborne particles from ever reaching your lungs.

There is a lining on the inside of your nasal cavity, which combined with the upper and lower respiratory tracts, contains special goblet cells whose main purpose is to secrete mucus. This mucus helps to moisten the air that you breathe as it comes into your body so that the air is as suitable for your body's internal environment as possible. On top of that, this mucus also traps particles, using the cilia to sweep them upwards and away from your lungs to go into your stomach. This not only helps to keep your lungs free from additional particles that shouldn't be there in the first place, but it also helps to move the particles into your stomach, where they will then be digested. While it may sound a little disgusting, it is a very effective way to keep particles that you inhale from ever getting trapped in your lungs.

When it comes to your lungs, they behave like little balloons. They do not have the power to inflate on their own but will easily inflate if there is air that is blown into them. While you can blow in to inflate them (which is going to be one of two different ways that cardiopulmonary resuscitation can be done), that probably will not happen in your regular daily life, as long as you are healthy. This means that for air to get into your lungs, you will need to inhale it and exhale it all on your own.

Now that you have just learned about how breathing actually works, as well as the entire process that happens with every breath that you take, you can surely see how beneficial it is to try to increase the efficiency of the entire process. If you can make even one aspect of this respiratory chain stronger and more efficient, it is going to have an overflow effect on every other one of the aspects involved.

For this reason, you should be excited to learn how optimizing your breathing can improve your life. Whether the benefits are for your mind, body, or spirit, when you can hone your breathing techniques, the benefits that you will see are going to surprise you. Here is everything that you need to know about breathing and how it can improve your life.

Chapter 2: How Breathing Can Improve Your Life

Stop reading for a second and take a deep breath. Didn't that make you feel much better than before you did it? Now think about that for just a second. All you did was to take one deep breath, and you immediately felt better than right before you took it. That's amazing, right? And doesn't this make you wonder what would happen if you did that multiple times per day? Or what if you were able to train yourself to take some deep breaths whenever a stressful situation arose?

This is exactly how getting your breathing under control and understanding can help you to make your life better. The impact of taking just a single deep breath can have on your body is tremendous, and the best thing about it is that this fantastic feeling is going to carry over into just about every aspect of your body. This means that when you can start breathing correctly, your life will be improved.

You may be wondering how you can start breathing to improve your life, and that's perfectly fine. With so much stuff going on in your busy life on a daily basis, it is easy to let your body handle something that it does automatically anyway (which is going to be breathing) without having to worry about spending even more of your valuable time 'fine-tuning' it. However, when you do fine-tune your breathing, the results it will have on you and every aspect of your life are going to be nothing short of life-changing.

I am going to tell you how you can begin to improve your breathing as quickly as right now and explain the benefits you can expect to receive from doing it. You may be thinking that you don't have time to work on improving your breathing, but what makes this so great is that you are only going to focus on incorporating one muscle right now: the diaphragm. Here is what you need to know about your diaphragm.

Your Diaphragm and You

Your diaphragm is one of the most important muscles in your body when it comes to breathing to improve your life. This is because the diaphragm is in charge of filling your lungs with air. It does this by acting as sort of a vacuum, sucking in as much air as it can through your respiratory system (which you just learned about above). On a side note, you should also know that your diaphragm aids your digestive system as well by massaging some of your internal organs. It works in conjunction with your pelvic floor to help your body create a stable core.

When you were born, you first used your diaphragm to breathe. If you watch any newborn baby try to breathe, you will notice that it is their belly that rises up and down, as this is how humans are supposed to be breathing all the time (what can't babies teach us?).

If you still need convincing, take a second and lie down on the floor, placing a couple of books onto your stomach. Now start to breathe regularly. You will notice that the books are going to move up and down. This is because your diaphragm is the muscle that does all the work of getting air into your lungs and not your chest or any other muscles that you may believe are involved.

As you grow from infancy into adulthood, somewhere along the line, you end up retraining the way you breathe, switching your main focus from the diaphragm and to the accessory breathing muscles. The accessory breathing muscles are the muscles within your rib cage, your neck, and even your shoulders. To further emphasize the point that you should be breathing from your diaphragm, the only time a baby uses their accessory breathing muscles to breathe is when they are sick or their breathing has been compromised in some way. Fast forward to adulthood, and the reason that you have changed the muscles involved with your breathing is mainly due to stress.

You may be wondering when or how this transfer of breathing occurred from your diaphragm to your breathing accessory muscles.

Whenever you breathe with your accessory muscles, you breathe the same way when your body goes into 'fight or flight' mode. Whenever you are in any type of stressful situation, the fight-or-flight response kicks in, and it will then change your breathing to deal with that situation. This is perfectly normal and exactly how the body was designed to deal with moments of stress. However, the one downside of this is that your body was only meant to be in fight or flight mode for a short period.

Think for just one second about your ancient ancestors and how their main concern was hunting and gathering.

They would go out on a hunt, chase down whatever animal they were hunting, or end up being confronted by a higher predator than they were. Once this happened, they would have to decide to stay and fight or try to run away. This was a decision that they had to make to ensure their survival. The physical work they had to do to get out of the stressful situation would be more than enough to counteract the fight-or-flight response. This would eventually lead their bodies to go back to homeostasis, and they would begin breathing with their diaphragm again.

Basically, the fight-or-flight response by the body shifts how you breathe from the diaphragm to the breathing accessory muscles. So, it stands to say that if you are always feeling stressed, your body is going to react by shifting how it breathes to use the breathing accessory muscles instead of just the diaphragm.

Fast forward to modern society—a sedentary lifestyle has pretty much become the norm, and the fact that most people are breathing with their accessory muscles starts to make sense. People are simply not moving anywhere near as much as they should be on a daily basis. On top of that, the stress that most people must deal with is not going to require very much physical activity to overcome either. Most of the stress that you undergo is actually more psychological than anything else. You have work, traffic, and financial stuff that you must deal with daily, which is also going to mean that this psychological stress is going to be more constant as well. This combination of living a sedentary lifestyle and constantly being under stress has retrained your body to change its breathing habits for the worse.

What's so Bad About Breathing Accessory Muscles?

If you constantly use your breathing accessory muscles to do all of your breathing, you are sending a signal to your body to constantly elicit a stress response. While you may feel that you are doing just fine, over time, you will notice that this continued state of stress response will lead you to have very poor posture, as well, and will have some horrible effects on some of your normal body functions. These effects can include:

- Having a posture that is hunched forwards
- Excessive neck pain due to carrying your head in a forward position
- A decrease in the efficiency of your digestive system
- A loss of your core stability
- A decrease in your body's thoracic stability
- When you are exercising, you may notice that you become fatigued very quickly (also referred to as early-onset fatigue)
- Your body has an increased amount of cortisol levels

While continuously breathing with your breathing accessory muscles can lead to some negative effects on your body, all is not lost! The good thing about your body and how you breathe is that you can retrain it to start doing it the correct way and making you feel great. Your diaphragm is one of the most dynamic muscles in your body. It can easily be trained, like every other muscle in your body. Here are some drills that you can start doing right now to reactive your diaphragm and the stress response of your body.

1. The Shoe Visual

Lay down on your back and place one of your shoes on your stomach and the other shoe on your chest. Inhale deeply through your nose, making sure that you push the shoe that is on your stomach up. Now exhale through your mouth or nose and watch as the shoe on your stomach starts to lower. Repeat this for a few minutes at a time. If you notice that the shoe sitting on your chest is the one that is rising and falling as you breathe, it means that you are using your accessory muscles, so try to focus on lifting the shoe on your stomach instead.

2. Ongoing Breathing

This can be done no matter whether you are standing up, sitting down, or even lying on your back. Place your hands right on top of your belly button. Now inhale through your nose, pushing your stomach and hands out. Exhale through your mouth or nose, making sure to feel your stomach naturally contract. Repeat for a few minutes at a time.

3. Crocodile Breathing

Start by lying down on your stomach. Place your forehead onto the back of your hands so that your neck is in a comfortable position. Start by inhaling through your nose, pressing your stomach onto the floor. When you do this, your stomach will not only push into the ground, but it will also expand and become wider as well—similar to how a crocodile breathes. Exhale through your mouth or nose, allowing your stomach to contract back to normal. Repeat this exercise a few minutes at a time.

Once you start doing these three simple breathing exercises, you will notice that your breathing will change in the sense that your diaphragm will be taking over your body's breathing functions more and more. As mentioned with the exercises, it is recommended that you start by doing at least one of the exercises for a few minutes every single day. Over time, you will begin to breathe like this without having to even think about it, no matter what situation you are in.

Now that you are familiar with how you should be breathing, you may be wondering what the benefits of correctly breathing are, in terms of improving your quality of life. Here are some of the ways that you can expect your life to get better when you are breathing the right way.

Breathing for a Better Quality of Life

When you can focus on your breath, it can be very beneficial for you as it will reduce the amount of stress that you are feeling, help you to burn more calories, help to improve your sex life, and much, much more. You would think that doing something so basic would be easy to get right, but as mentioned above, in today's society where you are always stressed out and are more than likely not getting enough regular exercise, most people are breathing all wrong. Breathing is one of the most important things that you will do all day long, but at the very same time, it is one of the things that you are going to not pay any attention to either. Because of this, breathing has become so dysfunctional that it is getting to the point where people think the dysfunctional way they are breathing is actually normal.

But you know the saying, "What you don't know can't hurt you," and that is exactly what is going on with breathing. When you can take a few minutes per day to fix the way that you breathe, you are going to be setting up your body to do some amazing things. For example, you can expect your anxiety to lessen, you will start getting much better sleep, and you will be able to exercise at a more intense level than you can now. What makes correcting your breathing so great is that these benefits are only going to be the tip of the iceberg! There are going to be many different benefits that you can expect your body to experience when you can get your breathing under control.

Here are some of the top ways that breathing can affect your body and improve your life for the better.

- **Breathing Helps to Relieve Stress**

Pretend that you are at work in the middle of a giant project, and nothing seems to be going well for you. While you are not going to notice it at all, your body's natural reaction is going to be to start taking short and shallow breaths. This is not good as it will increase the stress response in your body. If you do notice that this is happening, what you need to do is simply slow your breathing down to the rate of roughly five breaths per minute. This is not only going to reduce your stress levels, but it will also help stop anxiety in its tracks. So, the next time that you are feeling overwhelmed and stressed out, start breathing gently, but trying not to overfill your lungs, making sure that you are not forcing the air out of your lungs either when you exhale.

- **Try to Breathe Whenever You are in Pain**

No matter the conditions when you utilize breathing, it will help to lessen the amount of pain you are feeling. Whether that pain is from stubbing your toe, due to some type of chronic condition, or even if you are simply nursing a terrible headache, the way that you are breathing can help bring some relief. No matter the pain you are feeling, try to use a deeper and slower breathing technique, as it has been proven that this will actually increase your pain threshold. Now don't go and cut off a finger so that you can test this method, but by controlling your breathing, you will be able to help calm the amount of pain that you are feeling.

- **Breathing Will Help to Improve Your Sex Life**

Sexual dysfunction, performance anxiety, and many of the problems related to reaching orgasm can make people feel very anxious about having sex. So if you are dealing with one of these sexual conditions, you may want to try using some mindful breathing. This can make you more aware of the sensations that your body is feeling, as well as help track your sexual response. To do this, all you need to do is breathe in through your nose and out through your mouth. You can even add a mental count of a 'one-two' to relax a little bit more. If you are trying to take it to the next level, try imagining that you are breathing into your genitals. When you visualize it this way, it can help make you feel as though your genitals are actually coming alive and starting to activate. This is going to be a good thing as it can help you reach your orgasm faster and make it more powerful too!

- **Breathing When You Need to Concentrate**

Whenever you need to get down to business and get in the zone, try taking a few forceful and short breaths. Breathe in some air sharply, followed by exhaling that same air forcefully while you shout 'ha.' Try shooting for roughly 20 breaths a minute but limit this exercise to less than 5 minutes total. Just be sure that you close your office door before getting started, so you don't scare your coworkers. And if you suffer from high blood pressure, you may want to consider skipping this one altogether.

- **Breathing for Mindfulness**

Mindfulness is one of those words that has a lot of buzz around it these days. This is because the benefits of mindfulness include helping you to better control your emotions, which can improve your relationships and even reduce depression and anxiety. In case you were unfamiliar with mindfulness, it allows you to slow things down and start living in the moment, ideally meaning that you are going to enjoy your life that much more. To do this, you are going to want to focus all of your energy on your breathing, mainly focusing on how it is moving in and out of your body. This is also going to help you slow your breathing, as well as increase your overall feeling of calmness.

- **Breathing can Help You Run...During the Winter**

If you like to stay in shape, there is a very good chance that you run. But when the cold winter months move in, it can cause a huge hiccup in your workout plans. It is going to be very important for you to know that breathing through your nose while you are running during the winter months is going to give you a huge advantage. While it is more than likely going to be restricting and a bit more difficult in the beginning, this method will help to warm up the air prior to it reaching your lungs. This means that you are going to be getting much better oxygen consumption. If that is simply not in the cards, another method is to wear a scarf over your face and then breathe as you normally would when running. Whenever you breathe in any type of cold air, it is going to cause your airways to become constricted, so warming up the air is going to keep your airways feeling more relaxed. This means that you can expect to have a higher oxygen level within your body, helping your muscles get everything they need to continue performing.

- **Breathing to Spin (Exercise) Better**

If you are looking for a way to get into better shape faster, learn how to breathe through your nose first and then your mouth. However, being in the correct position to breathe is going to be even more important than the actual process of breathing. So be sure that you position yourself so that you're hinged at your hip (instead of rounding your back) when you lean over for the handlebars. This will provide your lungs with enough space to fill with all the air that they need. Do this and, all of a sudden, those big hills may seem just a little bit smaller.

- **Breathing to Lift Heavier Weights**

If you are looking to muster as much muscle power as you can, try inhaling during the eccentric (when you are lowering the weight) part of the lift, making sure to exhale while you perform the concentric (when you are lifting the weight) portion.

- **Breathing for a Stress-free Pregnancy**

The old school way of breathing with a 'hee-hee-hoo' type of breathing is best left for TV shows. If you are having some pregnancy pains, you want to go with something referred to as the 'cat and cow' method. To do this, get onto your hands and knees. You are then going to exhale and simultaneously round your back upwards (like a cat). Then inhale while forming an arch with the lower part of your back, ensuring that your tailbone is tipped outwards (like a cow). Make sure that both your inhales and exhales are nice and long, as it will help to keep your baby's and your blood pressure low.

- **Breathing to Fall Asleep Faster**

If you are one of the many people who have trouble falling asleep every night, the habits that you perform right before bed may be one of the contributing factors to your problem. To help alleviate this, try taking some slow, deep breaths as you climb into bed. This will help to relax your mind and body and calm you down as well.

- **Breathing Can Help with Your Asthma**

There are over 25 million people in the United States alone who suffer from asthma. Unfortunately for these people, there is no cure for asthma, meaning that if you do have it, you are going to need to be extra careful when it comes to managing it. This includes taking different medications, avoiding certain triggers, and making regular trips to the doctor's office. But studies have shown that doing certain breathing exercises can help to reduce the need to take the asthma medications that are regularly needed. Just be sure that you speak with your doctor if this is something that you are interested in trying for yourself.

To sum it up, breathing is something that you can do to change your life for the better. From the physical benefits to the calming effect it can have on you and the way that it can make your sex life that much better, breathing is something that you should spend a few minutes per day practicing. You spend time working on your muscles and increasing your endurance, so why not spend some time working on your breathing by strengthening your diaphragm as well? With all of the benefits that it can give you, it would be silly not to.

You know that breathing is a great tool that you can use to make your life better, but you keep hearing about things like CO_2 and that it relates to your oxygen levels in some way. You may have also heard that athletes are constantly getting CO_2 testing done, so does that mean that you need to get a CO_2 test as well? Here is what you are going to need to know about CO_2 and how you can use it to improve how you breathe.

Chapter 3: Testing and Improving Your CO2 Tolerance

If you are breathing, then you are also creating CO_2 (or carbon dioxide). In case you were not aware of what CO_2 is, it is a colorless and odorless gas that your body produces as a waste product from the oxygen utilization that was previously explained. Essentially, you breathe in oxygen, which your body can use to produce energy, and breathe out CO_2, which can cause you some serious harm if it is not removed from your body.

When oxygen is transferred from your blood cells to your body cells, CO_2 is transferred from your body cells to your blood cells. Your bloodstream then takes this CO_2 to your lungs so that it can be removed from your body when you exhale. So, every time you breathe in oxygen, you breathe out CO_2 without even thinking about it. This happens all day, every day and you are not conscious of the process. So, you may be wondering how exactly it is you test something like your CO_2 levels and why would you even want to measure it in the first place?

To answer that question, you must first understand that there are going to be two different measurements of CO_2. The first one is the levels of CO_2 in your blood, while the other test is a measurement of your CO_2 tolerance. Here is what you need to know about each of these tests and what they mean for you.

CO2 Blood Test

A CO2 blood test is often used in a series of tests that are referred to as an electrolyte panel. Since electrolytes help you balance the number of acids and bases that you have in your body, it is going to be very important to keep them at their optimal levels. Carbon dioxide is going to be a bicarbonate when it is in your body, meaning that it is going to be considered an electrolyte. It is important to know what your CO2 levels are in your bloodstream, as any type of imbalance can very easily lead you to suffer from several different diseases, including diseases in the lungs and kidneys, as well as high blood pressure.

To sum it up, a CO2 blood test will allow you to know how much CO2 you have in your body, as well as whether there is too much or too little of it. Depending on your levels, there can be several potential problems happening within your body. For example, if you have too much CO2 in your blood, it can mean that:

- You may have lung disease
- You may have Cushing syndrome, which is a disorder of your adrenal glands. They are in charge of helping to control your blood pressure, heart rate, and many other body functions as well. If you are suffering from Cushing syndrome, your adrenal glands are going to be producing too much cortisol, which is a hormone that can cause several different symptoms, including vision problems, muscle weakness, and even high blood pressure.
- You may be suffering from some type of hormonal disorder
- You may have a kidney disorder

- You may have alkalosis, which is a condition where your blood has too much base in it

If you have too little CO_2 in your blood, it is also bad. If this is the case, it means that:

- You may be suffering from Addison disease, which is going to be another disorder of your adrenal glands. With Addison disease, your adrenal glands are not going to be producing several different hormones at the rate that they should be, that including cortisol. If you do have this condition, it can cause you to develop a variety of symptoms that include dizziness, weakness, dehydration, and weight loss.
- You may have acidosis, which is a condition where your blood has too much acid in it.
- You may have ketoacidosis, which is essentially going to be a serious complication of both Type 1 and Type 2 diabetes, although quite rarely in type 2.
- You may go into shock
- You may have a kidney disorder

Keep in mind that if you do have a CO_2 blood test and your results come back saying that you are not in the 'normal' range, it does not mean that you will need to have immediate medical treatment for a disease. There may be other factors, such as certain medicines that you may be taking, which can alter the levels of CO_2 in your blood.

Now that you understand how important it is to make sure that you have the correct amount of CO_2 levels in your blood at any given time, how does that relate to breathing?

As mentioned earlier, your lungs and the air you exhale determine how efficiently your body can get rid of the excess CO_2 that it creates with every breath. If you are unable to get rid of CO_2 efficiently, it will start to build up in your bloodstream, as it won't have any way of being expelled from your body. This means that you will have a higher CO_2 level in your blood. This brings us to the next CO_2 test, which is called the CO_2 tolerance test.

CO2 Tolerance Test

A CO_2 tolerance test is basically a test that lets you know how efficiently you are using the oxygen that you breathe with every breath. You can then take the results from this test and use it to increase your breathing efficiency, meaning that you can expect to achieve better physical performance, and you can feel and be healthier than before. And unlike the CO_2 blood test that requires blood work and labs, the CO_2 tolerance test is only going to require that you have a stopwatch, which if you have bought a cell phone in the past 15 years, you should already have a stopwatch app built-in.

The whole point behind the CO_2 tolerance test is to find out how well you can tolerate carbon dioxide in your body, how well you are able to utilize the oxygen that you are breathing in, and even how well you can breathe. On top of that, the results are also going to be very closely correlated with how often and how easily you feel anxiety, how often you feel stressed out, and how susceptible you are to feeling as though you are not in control.

26

To take it a step further, when you have a higher CO_2 tolerance, it means that you will have a more efficient and optimized aerobic metabolism. This means that if you have a lower blood pH and a higher CO_2 blood level, your body is going to have a much easier time absorbing the oxygen that you are breathing. In other words, you are going to be maxing out your breathing rate before your body can utilize all of the oxygen that you breathe in. This is good because you will have a surplus of oxygen. However, if you have a poor CO_2 tolerance, it is going to be correlated with having poor breathing control. Essentially, if you are suffering from a low CO_2 tolerance, you can expect to struggle with physical activity much more than someone with a high CO_2 tolerance.

How to Take the CO2 Tolerance Test

As mentioned above, to take a CO_2 tolerance test, all you need is a stopwatch. Now don't worry, this is an extremely easy test to take, and you can even do it in the privacy of your own home. There are three steps to take this test, and it should take you no longer than a couple of minutes to complete, at the very most.

- **Step #1:** Take 4 very deep breaths, 1 breath every 5-10 seconds. Be sure that you are inhaling at a rate of 3-5 seconds for each breath, following this with a relaxed 5-10 second exhale. Once you have completed 1 breath, take a 1-second pause, and move onto the next inhale.

- **Step #2:** On the 4th breath (once your lungs are completely full), start the timer on your stopwatch and begin exhaling as slowly as you possibly can.

27

Try to stretch this exhale out as long as possible. On a side note, it may be helpful for you to close your eyes so that you can stay focused on this long exhale and feel more relaxed.

- **Step #3:** As soon as you run out of air or you need to take in a new breath, stop the timer.

Congratulations, you have just successfully performed a CO_2 tolerance test! Now the big question is, what do you do with the results you just recorded?

Since you remembered to keep track of how long you were able to exhale on the final breath, it is now time to interpret the results. Here is what the time it took you to exhale translates to in terms of your CO_2 tolerance levels.

CO_2 Tolerance Test Results Interpretation

To interpret your test results and see where you stand on the CO_2 tolerance test scale, match your time to the times that are listed below:

- **> 80 seconds = Elite**

You have an advanced pulmonary adaptation, can manage your stress exceptionally well, and have some excellent breathing control.

- **60-80 seconds = Advanced**

Your pulmonary system is healthy, you can manage stress relatively easily, and you have very good breathing control.

- **40-60 seconds = Intermediate**

This range means that you are able to improve your CO2 tolerance relatively quickly when you can focus on CO2 tolerance training.

- **20-40 seconds = Average**

You are more than likely going to be in a constant state of high anxiety and high stress. Your breathing mechanics require improvement as soon as possible.

- **< 20 seconds = Poor**

You suffer from extremely high stress and anxiety, you have a very poor pulmonary capacity, and you may be dealing with some sort of mechanical restriction issue.

Once you have your score and know where you stand as far as your CO2 tolerance goes, you should try to increase that score. It doesn't matter where you are on the scale. When you increase your CO2 tolerance, only good things are going to start happening to you and your body.

Why Increase Your CO2 Tolerance?

Whenever you exhale, you are going to be eliminating carbon dioxide from your body. This is because carbon dioxide is a waste product that is created by your body as a result of your body's cells turning oxygen and glucose into energy. With that being said, there are going to be some trace amounts of CO2 that do remain inside your body. But don't worry as this is a good thing.

As of right now, you have learned that CO2 is bad, but it is essential to the breathing process. In fact, it is a very necessary part of your respiratory system, even though it is always getting a bad rap. What is going to be bad though, would be the levels of CO2 in your body because the more CO2 in your body, the more signals your body will send that you need to breathe in more air. This is going to have nothing to do with the amount of oxygen that you are getting.

You can see this for yourself when you hold your breath. The longer that you can hold your breath, the greater your CO2 endurance will become. This is because CO2 is going to cause your blood vessels to dilate. On the other hand, oxygen will cause them to constrict. So, when you have a smaller percentage of CO2 in your blood, it is going to increase the amount of oxygenation in your blood and cells because the oxygen molecules can move more freely through the now dilated blood vessels.

To sum it up, when you have trace amounts of CO2 in your bloodstream, it is going to make the oxygenation of your body cells much easier, ultimately increasing the effectiveness of your entire body system.

Benefits of CO2 Tolerance

While it may seem that purposely trying to build up the amount of CO2 in your body may not be a great idea, you must keep in mind that even though over the long term it is not going to be a good thing, however, if practiced short term, it is going to be very beneficial to your body.

For example, hypoventilation, which is when you are consistently breathing at a weaker or slower state than normal, is going to increase the amount of acidity that is in your blood. Conscious breathing, however, is going to be about creating and finding a balance. When you can increase your CO_2 tolerance, your body will be able to handle this temporary imbalance prior to shifting back to normal.

For another example, consider your breathing during some type of athletic performance. While you are performing, you are going to be breathing more and using more oxygen, but you will be creating more carbon dioxide as well. If your CO_2 tolerance is on the lower side, you are going to start hyperventilating as your urge to breathe is going to be controlled by your body's response to the amount of CO_2 that is in your blood.

This same concept is also going to relate to inflammation, mental imbalance, anxiety, and stress as well. If you suffer from anxiety, you more than likely already know that hyperventilating is a somewhat common condition. It is the imbalance in your body that is increasing your urge to need to breathe. So, when you can build up and increase your CO_2 tolerance, it will help you to become much more comfortable in some of the uncomfortable situations that you may find yourself in.

Improving Your CO_2 Tolerance

All of the studies that have been done involving CO_2 tolerance have shown that you should increase it as much as you possibly can. Think of it like going to the gym, but for your breathing. When you go to the gym, you lift weights to get a stronger chest, back, legs, etc. However, not very many people even think about working out on their CO_2 tolerance, even though it has a direct relationship with the effectiveness of their workout when they are in the gym. With that being said, here are some simple exercises that you can start doing today in order to increase your CO_2 tolerance. The best thing about these exercises is that most of them don't require any equipment, and you can do them practically anywhere! So next time you in standing in line at the grocery store, why not give your CO_2 tolerance a little boost?

Exercise #1: Nasal Breathing While Working Out

If you can keep your mouth closed while you are exercising, it is going to force your body to start getting rid of the CO_2 it has at a much slower rate than you are used to. Try it out the next time you are exercising. Now it is going to make it somewhat harder for you to train, but at the very same time, it is going to put your pulmonary system to work at maximum efficiency.

Exercise #2: Counted Breathing Exercises

Find a quiet place where you can sit down uninterrupted for 10-15 minutes. Set a timer for about 10 minutes, shut your eyes, and then use the breath to count the guidelines listed below. Try to breathe with the very same pattern repetitively until the timer expires.

- **If you are a beginner:** Try to exhale at a rate that is slightly longer than your inhale. A great starting place is going to be to try to inhale for a count of 8 and exhale for a count of 10.

- **If you are intermediate:** You are still going to want to exhale for a longer amount of time than you inhale, but this time utilizing a breath-hold after every inhale. Try starting with a count of 8 on the inhale, a breath-hold count of 4, and then an exhale for a count of 10.
- **If you are advanced:** Exhale for a much longer time than your inhale, utilizing a breath-hold after each exhale. Try inhaling for a count of 8, followed by an exhale of a count of 10. After your exhale is complete, try a breath-hold count of 4 before taking your next inhale.

Exercise #3: Hold Your Breath

One of the best ways that you can increase your CO_2 tolerance is to simply hold your breath. To do this, simply take an inhale and hold it for as long as you can. As soon as you are no longer able to hold that breath, exhale it in a slow, controlled manner. After your exhale has been completed, repeat the entire process over again. Repeat this for 5-10 minutes at a time.

When it comes to your CO_2 tolerance, it is going to be very important in terms of helping you stay calm and prevent your body from going into 'panic' mode. The higher your CO_2 tolerance, the more oxygen you are going to be able to get out of the same amount of air that you breathe. This is why it is crucial for you to increase this tolerance to be the best that it can be. The number of benefits that more oxygen can provide you with has been explained in the earlier chapters in this book, so you already know their importance (do you need to be reminded of the better sex?). Since all of the aforementioned exercises to increase your CO_2 tolerance can be done in the privacy of your home, while you are at the office, as you sit in traffic, or just about anywhere else you can think of, there is really no excuse for you to not start practicing them today. When you do, things are only going to get better!

If you have tried any of the previously mentioned breathing exercises, you have just done what is known as 'breathwork.' Breathwork is when you practice or work on your breathing through certain breathing techniques. Here is what you need to know about breathwork, the good, the bad, and the ugly.

Chapter 4: Breathwork — What You Need to Know

For hundreds and even thousands of years, humans have been practicing controlled breathing to help reduce their stress, increase their overall alertness, and even give their immune system the boost that it needs to keep illness away. While several different breathing practices have been used for centuries, it was only recently that science started to provide the research and evidence that the benefits of these ancient practices are real. Several studies have found that when you do start a breathing routine regularly, it has the power to help you reduce problems such as insomnia, anxiety, depression, post-traumatic stress disorder; it can even increase your ability to pay attention for longer periods.

In ancient times, the art of breathing was referred to as meditating, but in recent years it has become known as breathwork. Here is exactly what you need to know about breathwork before you get started, as well as what science has to say about its effectiveness.

What Exactly is Breathwork?

Breathwork is considered a special type of exercise that you can use to manipulate your breathing depth and rate. The main goal of practicing breathwork is to bring more awareness to your breath. This is done by providing benefits that are similar to meditation. As previously mentioned, your breathing and how effectively your body can utilize the oxygen it inhales is going to make a huge difference in just about every aspect of your body: physically, mentally, and even physiologically. So, when you can increase how efficiently your body uses the oxygen you breathe each day, you will be able to reap the benefits that come along with it.

For most people who practice breathwork, they are going to do so for anywhere between 20 minutes to one full hour. This is going to include a very sustained and rhythmic technique, but don't be scared off by that kind of time commitment. If you are just starting in breathwork and only looking to test the waters, there will be several other breathwork techniques that you can do which have a much shorter time commitment. These will be explained shortly. With that being said, you must keep in mind that you are only going to get out of it what you put into it, so the bigger the investment you put into your breathwork, the bigger and better the benefits you will have.

For those who are already practicing breathwork (and for those who are curious what they should expect after they get started), it has been described by some as a feeling of tingling sensations that radiate throughout the entire body, followed by feelings of extreme clarity and alertness, as well as an improved mind-body connection.

The Different Types of Breathwork

When it comes to the different types of breathwork that you can practice, there will be many different ones to choose from. Some of them range from being more basic and something that you can easily do at home or in your office at work, while others are going to require that you find a breathwork practitioner to teach you that particular practice. It is all going to depend upon your main goal with breathwork and your level of commitment.

You will find that some breathwork practices are rooted in various yogic traditions, including Pranayama or the movement and breath sequences that are used in Kundalini Yoga. Yet other practices of breathwork are entirely secular, and the main reason they were developed is to help you heal your mind and body; oftentimes, they are used to help you withstand some type of extreme physical condition.

While there will be several types of breathwork practices that you can try, the trick is not just choosing one and forcing yourself to use it, but rather to try several and decide which one is the best for you. If you simply choose one breathwork practice and force yourself to do it even though you are not necessarily enjoying it, there is a very high probability that you will not stick with it. On the other hand, if you take the time to try three or four different breathwork practices, you will be more likely to find one that best fits your needs and that you enjoy doing. Once you have found the practice that you enjoy the most, you will be much more likely to stick with it, meaning that the benefits that come along with it will be achieved much sooner. Think of it like starting an exercise regimen or going on a diet; if you start an exercise program or diet that you simply do not like or enjoy, your fail rate is going to be astronomical. However, if you find that you enjoy doing Zumba or eating a keto diet, you will be much more motivated to stay with it, meaning that you can expect to achieve a much better result in a much shorter period.

No matter which type of breathwork practice you decide to try, do your best to keep an open mind and remember that if you are simply not feeling one specific breathwork practice, it doesn't mean that you won't like a different one. So do your best to try out a few different breathwork practices at first, eventually deciding upon the one that you would like to focus on the most.

What You Can Expect After Starting Breathwork

If you are this far into this eBook, you have already read about the different benefits that deep breathing can provide you with. In fact, even a few deep breaths at a time can lower your blood pressure, drop your cortisol levels, and even increase your parasympathetic tone. But when it comes to breathwork, the benefits are going to be slightly different. When you practice formal breathwork, they are going to exert even more positive effects on your body and your mind, almost working in a different and somewhat opposite direction. Here are some of the main health benefits that you can expect to see after you have started practicing breathwork.

- **It Alkalizes the pH of Your Blood**

When you practice breathwork, you are going to notice that there will be some physiological changes that occur. These are going to be caused by a shift in your blood's pH levels, just like the ones that follow hyperventilation. Essentially, you are going to be putting your body into a state of 'respiratory alkalosis,' which happens when you have a sustained and rhythmic breathing pattern. While there is not much known about respiratory alkalosis, recently, the anesthesiology field was able to make huge strides in understanding what is happening with your body when it occurs.

As was described earlier, your body is going to inhale to get the oxygen from the breath and exhale to get rid of the CO_2 waste out of your body. When you start to take a faster breath, you will start to get rid of more of the CO_2 that is in your body. Since CO_2 is an acidic molecule, the more that you can get out of your body using hyperventilating, the more acid you are effectively going to be getting out of your blood. This means that your blood's pH will start to become more alkaline (this is where the term respiratory alkalosis comes from). When this happens, there will be a couple of different benefits that you can expect to see.

- **You May Notice an Increase in Your Muscle Tone**

Once your blood's pH has become more alkaline, there are a few different things that you can expect to happen. First, the calcium ions that are floating around throughout your bloodstream will start to go into hiding. They do this by binding to the larger proteins known as albumin that is present in your blood. Once this occurs, your body will then be in a temporary low-calcium state, which is then going to increase the firing in both your motor and sensory neurons. This 'artificially' low blood calcium is now going to start manifesting itself in your neurological system; this will be experienced through tingling sensations, your smooth muscles contracting, and an increase in your muscle tone. If you have ever been to a breathwork class that has left you feeling as though you were not able to move your mouth, you will know exactly how this feels.

- **There is an Anti-inflammatory Effect**

When you are in hyperventilation, the neurons inside your autonomic nervous system are going to fire much more, which means your body is going to release an excess of epinephrine into your system. This is going to be the very same thing that many people refer to as 'adrenaline.' When this influx of epinephrine occurs, it causes your immune system to start increasing its anti-inflammatory response. This means that your pro-inflammatory activity will then become dampened. What all of this means is that when you begin a breathwork routine that you do regularly, you are going to have a much less severe inflammatory response when exposed to bacterial toxins than those who are not practicing a breathwork routine.

- **Your Mood will be Elevated**

If you are regularly doing breathwork, you are already more than likely familiar with the 'high' feeling that can occur during your hyperventilation and state of respiratory alkalosis. When you have an increased blood pH, it is going to decrease the amount of oxygen that is delivered to your body tissues. This is going to be more commonly referred to as the Bohr Effect. Happening within the first minute that you start to hyperventilate, the vessels in your brain will begin to constrict, ultimately reducing the blood flow to your brain. By reducing the blood flow to your brain, you are also going to be reducing the amount of oxygen that your brain is receiving, oftentimes to the tune of around 40%. This effect is more than likely going to be responsible for all of the different feelings of happiness and wellbeing that those who practice breathwork are experiencing. What this all means is that when you practice breathwork regularly, you are essentially going to be getting an all-natural high at the very same time.

With all of the benefits that breathwork has to offer you, there is a very good chance that you are ready to get started! But at the very same time, it can be intimidating and often scary to simply jump into a new lifestyle without really knowing what to expect. With that being said, here is everything that you will need to know before getting started with your breathwork.

What to Know Before You Start a Breathwork Routine

If you have never done any type of breathwork before, you may have some worries about whether you will enjoy doing it, whether it is safe, and likewise. With those concerns being said, what you need to know is that yes, breathwork is generally 100% safe. It is a very enjoyable and well-tolerated activity, so most people who try it end up enjoying and sticking with it. While it is going to be like everything else in that it is not for everyone, those who stand to benefit the most from breathwork will be those who are suffering from any type of autoimmune disease, those looking to improve their health and wellbeing, and anybody who is overwhelmed and feels stressed out more often than not.

However, even though you know that there are a ton of benefits that you can reap from doing a regular breathwork routine, there will be a few different circumstances where you may not want to attempt any type of breathwork. While these situations seldom occur, they do happen. So, if you are suffering from any type of cardiac arrhythmia (including having a very slow heart rate), you have a history of heart blockage, or you are taking a certain type of antipsychotic medication, it is highly recommended that you do not attempt any type of breathwork practices or routines. Any conditions other than those should be absolutely fine to get started with a regular breathwork routine. If you are unsure or just want to double-check to make sure that it is safe for you to start a breathwork routine, speak with your doctor about what it is you are trying to do and let them know what your plan is. This way, they will be informed about your new breathwork venture and will be able to monitor your results as your progress moves forward.

On a side note, while breathwork is generally safe for just about everybody to do, there are some practices of breathwork that can leave you feeling dizzy, cause slight chest pain, make it feel as though your heat is pounding, and induce you to start hyperventilating. While these side-effects are going to depend on different factors, such as your current fitness level, the type of breathwork you are doing, and the level of effort that you are putting into it, they are side-effects that you should know about before you get started with any type of breathwork routine. But when you start at the level that is suitable for you, you will more than likely not have to worry about any of these side-effects at all.

To sum up what you should know about breathwork:

- It involves manipulating how you breathe to alter your breathing rate, ultimately affecting how you feel and how your body is temporarily going to function.
- There are many different types of breathwork practices that you can do. While some are going to be more basic, and you will be able to do them in the comfort of your own home, others are going to require that you seek a special practitioner to help guide you through.
- There are many benefits that you can expect to receive from doing a regular breathwork routine, the most popular being a reduction in your stress and anxiety levels, a reduced amount of inflammation, and an alkalized pH level in your blood.
- You should always spend a few minutes and speak with your doctor prior to getting started with any type of breathwork routine. If you have a history of high blood pressure, are currently taking some sort of antipsychotic medication, or are suffering from any other type of cardiovascular disease, you may want to wait to get started with any type of breathwork.

Now that you are more than familiar with just about everything breathwork, except for the actual breathwork that you should be doing, there are certain situations where breathwork can help. Here is how you should be using breathwork for certain situations.

Chapter 5: How to Use Breathwork to Improve Your Focus in the Most Stressful of Situations

Breathwork is going to have many different benefits that you can achieve from it. What makes breathwork even more special is the fact that you can use it to help calm yourself in many different situations. No matter where you are, what you are doing, or what the situation may be, you can use breathwork to help calm yourself and get a better grasp on the situation that you are facing. Using breathwork to help defuse things such as a stressful situation is not a technique you can learn overnight. The only real way that you can ensure that your breathwork techniques are going to work when you began to feel overstressed is by practicing them before you need to use them. Think of breathwork as karate. Karate is a great tool to have when somebody attacks you, but if you have not practiced any karate before being attacked, it is more than likely not going to really serve you with any purpose. The same is true with breathwork. If you are already practicing it, then when you do need it, the results are going to be amazing. But if you have not been practicing, there is a good chance that you are not going to attain your desired outcome. Essentially, practice your breathwork if you want it to work for you when you need it.

When you can practice your breathwork in advance, the breathing techniques you use will help to restructure how your brain works, trigger the physiological process that is responsible for improving your health, and even help shape your mind so that it is much more capable of experiencing peace and happiness.
While you can get started with breathwork anytime that you want to, you must first prepare yourself to embark on this very transformational journey. This means that you will need to get ready to experience both an inward and outward transformation. No matter what, be sure that you always remember that you are doing this to help make yourself the best version of you that you can be. There is a very good chance that you are going to be walking this path alone, and not everybody is going to be supportive or even understand what you are doing. But when you stay true to yourself and realize you are doing this to become as healthy as you can possibly be, you will have no problem incorporating breathwork and benefiting from everything it has to offer. That aside, here is how you can use breathwork to improve your focus in the most stressful of situations.

Establish Some Type of Daily Routine

When it comes to practicing your breathwork so that you can make it work for you in even the most stressful of situations, you will need to create some type of daily routine to allow yourself to practice. To do this, you should start by choosing a time of the day when you will have some peace and quiet, ideally not being disturbed by anything, including any type of other responsibilities that you or your family may have. For many people, this means doing their breathwork early in the morning or later in the evening after everybody else has gone to sleep. On a side note, however, if you have decided that you are going to do your breathwork after the rest of your family has gone to sleep, you may have to deal with your own sleepiness as well. No matter what the time of day may be, make sure that you can invest it into your breathwork while not being disturbed.

Once you have carved out a little bit of time to dedicate to your breathwork, the next thing you need to do is to find the perfect location. Try selecting one of the quieter corners of your home, making sure that you can dim the lights. This area should be very organized and free from any potential distractions or clutter. If you have a clock that ticks, it is going to be more annoying than you could have imagined while you are practicing your breathwork, so try to use a clock that has illuminated numbers if you are practicing after dark. Once you get some experience with our breathwork though, you will have an understanding of how much time has passed and will only need to use the clock every now and then. Speaking of clocks, in the beginning, they are going to be a very important part of your breathwork. If you are not using a clock to keep track of your time, there is a very good chance that you would simply get up when sitting becomes uncomfortable. This is something that is definitely ok to do, but it will also be very counterproductive in terms of developing your focus.

To develop your ability to sit and practice your breathwork and concentration for a longer period of time, try sitting with both of your legs very loosely crossed, or even in a kneeling position if this position is more comfortable. Make sure that you use a firm cushion or a couple of folded blankets that are high enough for you to let your knees slightly dropped down. If you need more stability, try using crossed-leg positions, as this is going to give you a solid 'tripod' type base. If you find that this position is not working for you, you can always try to sit on the edge of a chair, making sure to place your feet flat on the floor and have them crossed at your ankles.

A lot of breathwork is going to be about finding the positions you are comfortable being in for a period of time, so you may want to experiment with some type of back support or even a soft couch. The only downside to this is that there is the potential to cause you drowsiness, which would in turn make doing your breathwork much more difficult. You are simply going to need to try different things until you find what works for you. For example, if you will be doing your breathwork in a room that is normally cooler, you may want to use a shawl and drape it around your shoulders. The idea here is to be warm, not to be hot. When you do utilize a shawl, it will double as a sense of protection and comfort, and that will be an added bonus.

Be sure that the location you decide to do your breathwork in is free from insects or bugs. If there are some in the space, be sure that you compassionately remove them from the room, moving them to an outside area. The last thing you are going to want to deal with while focusing on your breathwork is a buzzing fly or mosquito. Also, be sure to close any windows and turn off any technology that may potentially distract you from what you are doing. After you have found the perfect spot to practice your breathwork, you can now get started with your breathwork practice.

To get started, go to the comfortable sitting position that you have already found, fold your hands into your lap (or you can also rest them on your knees if you would like), and close your eyes. Now that you are all ready to start practicing your breathwork, it can help you when you are overstressed.

Focus on Feeling Your Breath

Now that you are in the perfect position to practice your breathwork, you should always start your training session with a very quiet and calm mind. Once you feel as though you are ready, try to direct all of your attention toward your breathing. At this point, there is no need to control your breath, but you should just put all of your focus on it. There is no need to do any type of deep breathing, breath control, or even alteration of your breathing pattern. Being aware of your breath is not an actual breathing exercise but more of an observation that you are making on how you regularly breathe.

When you inhale, focus on feeling your breath flow over every part of your nostrils and upper lip. Make sure you notice the cool temperatures or the slight stinging sensation that you feel inside your nose. On the exhale, take note of how your breath feels as it exits your nose; the warm air flowing out of your body, and touching the small area of skin that is the opening of your nostrils. Try to do this for the next 20 minutes, making sure that you are continuously aware of all your inhales and exhales, taking note of how they softly touch your skin around your nostrils and the warm or cool sensations that accompany them.

Your main goal in this breathwork is going to be developing the ability to concentrate on your breath without becoming distracted. While this is going to take some time to accomplish, every extra minute that you can continue this exercise is going to be a huge win on your part. Until you can make your mind sensitive and calm, there is a very good chance that you will not be able to feel the breath's touch. If this is the case, simply breathe a little bit harder until you do feel it. As soon as you feel it, immediately go back to your regular breathing, and identify whether you can still feel your breath or not. Repeat this process until you are successful. Even if you don't feel anything, when you continue to focus on the area right below your nostrils, you are eventually going to feel the almost imperceptible touch of air.

This technique is going to require you to observe and feel the natural and soft touch of your respirations. Natural breath is essentially going to mean your ordinary, normal breath that you take every single day. There will be times where you will find your natural breath is shallow and rapid, while there will be other times that your breath is deep and long. There will be other times that your breathing is going to be on the erratic side, while still others it will be rhythmic. You will even have times that you have a stuffy nose, meaning that your breath is going to be noisy or strained. The ultimate thing that you will need to remember is that your main focus with breathwork is always going to be your normal, natural breath and being aware of it.

Observe Your Normal, Natural & Ordinary Breath

While there is a number of different breathwork exercises you can do in order to reduce your stress and anxiety, all of these exercises will get the job done. It does not matter if you prefer to use the Pranayama technique, belly breathing, or even controlled breathing; you know what works best for you and should always use that technique. There are also going to be those who will visualize a white light while they breathe, using this breath to energize and heal different parts of your body. While these breathing methods are all going to be very similar, they are not quite going to be the same as this method.

To fully understand the difference between the methods, it will be very helpful to set aside all other breathing techniques while you learn this particular one. If you are not able to separate the different techniques from each other, there is a very good chance that you will mix them up and compromise any of the results that you are trying to achieve. It will be very important to make sure that you practice the breathwork exactly as instructed. This will allow you to go back to some of the other breathwork methods and understand the difference between them.

When you have breath awareness, it will provide you with a way to observe reality and be objective about it. The entire goal of breathwork is to allow you to take in a situation and not react in a negative way. In fact, this is the exact way that breathwork can help you control your stress and anxiety in just about any situation. When you can use breathwork to help control how you feel in the moment, you are essentially going to be able to eliminate any type of stress that may have arisen under any other circumstances. Essentially, when you start observing your regular breathing due to the breathwork that you have done, it is going to eliminate the stress that certain situations cause, meaning that you will still be able to experience that event, but in a much calmer and more 'aware' way.

Be Aware of Each and Every Breath that You Take

With this technique of breathwork, you are actually not going to be following each breath you take. Instead, you are going to focus all of your attention on that small area of skin that is located right below your nose. Breath awareness is how aware you are of your breath as it passes over this particular spot.

The smaller the spot you are able to focus on, the more aware of your breath and the sharper your focus will become. While this may sound easy to do, you would be surprised to discover that you may actually have some difficulty with it. If this is the case, try focusing on a larger area at first. As you are able to increase your focus on this larger area, the next step is to make the area a little smaller. Continue repeating this process of creating a smaller and smaller area to focus on as you get more comfortable with your breathwork.

If you are unable to feel your breath on this particular spot while you are inhaling, try taking some harder breaths until you are able to feel it. As soon as you detect it, go back to your regular, natural breathing. As long as you are able to fix all of your attention on this one area where you should be feeling every breath, your mind is going to naturally become more alert and sensitive.

It will not be long until you are able to feel even the lightest of your breaths. However, if you are distracted or your mind is preoccupied with something, it may be hard to feel your breaths touch on this particular area. If that is the case, the last thing that you are going to want to do is to worry. Simply continue to focus on this same area of skin that is right under your nose. There is a very good chance that you will feel your skin itching, throbbing, vibrating, tickling, or even stinging, but this is okay. While these sensations are not going to be caused by your breathing, they can be used as a tool to keep you focused on that area until you are able to feel your breath there. Be sure that you stay focused on continuing your natural breathing without missing even one breath. Try to pay attention to how many breaths you have taken until you notice that your mind has started to wander but do your best to avoid counting. The reason for this is that when you count your breaths, counting can become a very big distraction, as it will take away from your ability to focus on your breathing. If you are just starting with this particular breathwork technique, it may only be 6 or 7 breaths until you notice that your mind has started to wander. As soon as you do notice that your mind has started to wander, all you need to do is bring it back to focusing on your breath. The more you practice this technique, the longer you will be able to focus your mind on your breathing. While in the beginning, it is going to be difficult to focus, the more that you practice, the better you will get, and the easier this practice will become.

The best way that you can utilize breathwork to help you stay calm during a very stressful situation is going to be to have already started with a breathwork routine. This is going to be the best way that you will be able to help calm yourself and relieve some of the stress and anxiety that you are starting to feel. However, what if you are in a stressful situation and you have not yet started any type of breathwork routine? You are still going to need to calm down but will not have the breathwork knowledge that you need to do so. If that is the case, there are going to be several different types of breathwork exercises that you can do at that moment to help you calm yourself. Here is how you can use some simple breathwork exercises whenever you feel as though your anxiety and stress levels are starting to go into overload.

Breathwork Exercises to do When You Feel Anxious and Stressed Out

Feeling as though you are unable to breathe when you are experiencing stress or anxiety can be a very frightening thing to have to deal with. This is going to be even more frightening if you are unaware of how to defuse the situation and calm yourself down. Luckily for you, however, there are going to be some breathing techniques that you can do to help you alleviate some of the symptoms that you are experiencing and help you feel better almost immediately.

Here are some of the different breathing exercises that you can use to keep yourself calm and basically hit the 'reset' button in any situation.

- **Try to Lengthen Your Exhale**

The simple act of taking a deep inhale is not always going to help calm you down. In fact, when you take a deep breath, it is more than likely going to link to your sympathetic nervous system, which is the system that controls your fight or flight response. This means that when you do take a deep breath, you are essentially telling your body to start activating the fight or flight mechanism in your body. This is not going to do you any good when you are trying to calm down over a stressful situation.

Instead, you want to focus on your exhale, which is going to be linked to your parasympathetic nervous system. This system will be responsible for influencing your body's ability to stay calm and relaxed.

When you take too many deep breaths in a short period of time, it can actually lead you to start hyperventilating, which is bad as it will decrease the amount of oxygen-rich blood that is going to be flowing to your brain. If you do feel as though you are starting to drown under too much stress or anxiety, it is going to be much easier to breathe too much, which can potentially end in you hyperventilating, even if you are trying to do the exact opposite of that. Here Is what you should do other than taking extra breaths when you do start to feel overwhelmed with stress.

1. Before you do what you naturally want to do and take a big breath of air, try to let out an extra thorough exhale instead. Focus on pushing all the air out of your lungs, following that by allowing your lungs to work their magic and refill on their own.
2. After that, you are going to want to spend a bit more time exhaling than inhaling. For example,

you can try to inhale for a count of four but exhale for a count of six.

3. Repeat this process for the next two to five minutes.

The best part about this exercise is that you can do it just about anywhere, meaning that if there is any situation that is starting to stress you out, you are prepared to handle it with your breathwork. You can even do this when you are sitting, standing, or lying down.

- **Do Abdominal Breathing**

When you breathe with your diaphragm (using the muscle that sits right beneath your lungs discussed in-depth earlier), which is also commonly referred to as 'belly breathing,' it can help you reduce the amount of work that your body must do in order for you to breathe. To start breathing from your diaphragm, try the following breathing technique:

1. For this breathing technique, you are going to want to be as comfortable as possible, meaning that you should find a space that allows you to lie down, ideally on the floor or your bed, using pillows to rest your head and knees on. If that is not plausible, you can always find a comfortable chair to sit in, making sure that your head, shoulders, and neck are relaxed and your knees are bent.
2. Next, place one of your hands right underneath your rib cage, and place your other hand over your heart.
3. Began to inhale and exhale, trying to do both through only your nose. Make sure that you are

noticing how, or if, your stomach and chest are moving as you continue to breathe in and out.

4. Are you able to isolate how you are breathing in order to bring air even deeper into your lungs? What about the opposite of this? Are you able to breathe so that your chest is moving more than your stomach is moving?

Ideally, you are eventually going to be able to get to a point where your stomach is moving with every breath you take, meaning that your chest will not be moving. This is why this particular method is known as abdominal breathing or belly breathing. While you will most likely need to practice abdominal breathing before you are able to really utilize its effectiveness in any stressful situation, there are going to be some tips that you can use to master this type of breathing much quicker.

To practice your belly breathing:

1. Lie or sit down exactly as was described above.
2. Place one of your hands on your chest and the other hand somewhere that is right above your belly button.
3. Take a breath through your nose, making sure to take note that your stomach is rising. Your chest should remain still and not move at all.
4. Purse your lips and began to exhale through your mouth. During this exhale, try to engage the muscles of your stomach, helping to push out the air until you have none left.
5. Repeat this process for several minutes.

If you really want this type of breathing to become automatic so that you can do it whenever you are in a stressful situation and you need to calm down, you are going to need to practice it daily. For starters, you can try doing belly breathing four to five times per day for up to 10 minutes per session.

On a side note, if you have not been breathing with your diaphragm in the beginning, you may find that you get tired fairly quickly. However, the more you practice belly breathing, the better you will become, and the easier it will get.

- **Practice Breath Focus**

Whenever your deep breathing is slow and focused, it is going to help you reduce the amount of stress and anxiety that you may be feeling. For this technique, you will either lie down or sit in a place that is quiet and comfortable. Once you are in position, you should:

1. Make a note of how it feels when you are inhaling and exhaling normally. Take a moment to mentally scan your body and how it feels in the moment. You may find that there is some tension that you had not been aware of.
2. Now take a very slow, deep breath, making sure that you inhale only through your nose.
3. Notice how your upper body and your stomach are expanding.
4. Exhale your breath using the method most comfortable for you (which is going to be either your nose or your mouth), sighing if you feel like it.

5. Repeat this process for several minutes, making sure that you are paying attention to how your stomach is rising and falling.
6. Next, choose a word that you can focus on, vocalizing that word during every exhale. Some sample words are going to be 'calm' or 'safe,' as these are going to be words that are effective at helping you to calm down.
7. When you inhale, try to imagine it as a wave that is washing over your entire body.
8. When exhaling, imagine that your exhaled breaths are only there to serve one purpose: to carry any negative and upsetting thoughts or energy out of your body and away from you.
9. If you find that you become distracted during this breathing technique, gently bring your attention back to your breathing and the words that you were using to help relieve your stress levels.

Try to practice this technique for a minimum of 10, but upwards of 20 minutes per day whenever you can. If you do, you will find that you are going to experience much less stress and anxiety throughout your day, meaning that this breathwork practice is not only working but that your day is less stressful as well.

- **Try doing Equal Breathing**

Another type of breathing that you can use when you feel as though you are becoming overstressed or overwhelmed with anxiety is going to be one that stems from the ancient practice of Yoga that is known as Pranayama Yoga. This practice is also known as equal breathing. What makes equal breathing so great is the fact that you can practice it while you are either sitting or lying down. No matter what position you decide to practice this type of breathing in, just be sure that you are comfortable in that position. Once you are comfortable, you should:

1. Close your eyes and start paying attention to how you are normally breathing for several different breaths.
2. Next, start to slowly count 1-2-3-4 as you are inhaling through your nose.
3. Once you have completed your inhale, start to exhale following the very same four-second count.
4. As you continue to inhale and exhale, try to be mindful of the feelings of both emptiness and fullness that you feel in your lungs.

As you continue to practice equal breathing, you may find that your second count is going to vary. If this is the case, you have no need to be alarmed. As long as you are able to keep your inhales and your exhales the same, you are doing the breathing work correctly and have nothing to worry about.

- **Resonant Breathing**

Also referred to as coherent breathing, resonant breathing will help you to calm your anxiety and get your entire body into a very relaxed state. To do resonant breathing, you should:

1. Lie down in a quiet place where you can relax and close your eyes.

2. Start to gently breathe in through your nose, making sure that you keep your mouth closed for a total of six seconds worth of inhaling.
3. Be sure that you don't over-fill your lungs, making sure that they do not become too full of air.
4. Slowly exhale for six seconds, allowing your breath a chance to completely leave your body in a very slow and gentle manner. Whatever you do, try your best to not force your breath out of your body.
5. Repeat these steps for the next 10 minutes.
6. Once you have completed 10 minutes of this style of breathing, allow yourself a few extra minutes to simply be still and focus on how your body is feeling in that moment.

Resonant breathing is going to be something that you can do whenever you start to feel stressed and need a way that you can help diffuse the situation. While you don't have to rely solely on this method of breathing, when you partner this with the other types of breathwork techniques mentioned here, you will have all the tools that you need in order to calm yourself in any situation that you may get into.

- **Try Practicing Yogic Breathing (Pranayama Breathing)**

Unless you live in a cave, you have more than likely heard of a special health and wellness practice that is known as Yoga. One of the main things that Yoga focuses on is breathing, as Yoga has used breathing since it was originally created. Essentially, it is safe to say that at the heart of every type of Yoga is going to be breathing variations.

One particular form of Yoga known as Pranayama is going to include multiple breathing variations that will help you to relieve both stress and anxiety. While some of these methods will include a lengthened exhale or even equal breathing (both of which have been explained earlier), they also utilize what is known as 'lion's breath' and alternate between nostril breathing, which is also going to be known as Nadi Shodhana.

- **Lion's Breath**

Lion's breath is a breathing exercise where you exhale your breath in a very forceful manner. If you want to try lion's breath, you need to:

1. Get into a comfortable kneeling position, making sure that you cross your ankles and rest your butt on your feet. If this ends up not being comfortable enough for you to sit for an extended amount of time, you can always sit with your legs crossed instead.
2. Next, bring both of your hands to your knees, making sure that you stretch out your arms, as well as your fingers.
3. Take a deep breath in through your nostrils, making sure that your mouth is closed.
4. Begin to exhale through your mouth, putting an emphasis on vocalizing the word 'ha.'
5. While you are exhaling, you should open your mouth as wide as you possibly can so that you are able to stick your tongue out, trying your best to

stretch it downwards towards your chin as far as it is able to go. Essentially, you are going to try to touch your tongue to your chin.

6. Start to focus on the middle of your forehead (also referred to as your third eye) or the tip of your nose while you are completing your exhale.
7. Relax your face and then repeat this process, starting with the inhale.
8. Do this breathing technique up to six times in a row, making sure that you change how your ankles are crossed as soon as you get to the halfway point (meaning that you need to switch the cross of your ankles after 3 of these breaths).

- **Alternating Nostril Breathing**

When it comes to alternating nostril breathing, you will sit in a very comfortable, quiet place that will allow you to focus. Once you have found this spot, you will try to lengthen your spine while simultaneously opening your chest as much as you possibly can.

1. Take your left hand and place it in your lap, raising your right hand. Next, take the middle and pointer fingers on your right hand and place them onto your forehead, right between your eyebrows. Now close your eyes, inhaling and exhaling through only your nose, meaning that your mouth is going to need to remain closed during this entire process.
2. Take your thumb (from your right hand) and use it to close your right nostril, inhaling very slowly through your left nostril.
3. Once you have inhaled, pinch your nose closed using your right ring finger and thumb, meaning

that you are going to be holding your breath for a quick moment.

4. Keep your left nostril closed with your right ring finger and remove your thumb from the right nostril so that you can exhale all your air, waiting a moment before you begin your next inhale.
5. Inhale slowly through your right nostril.
6. Use your fingers to pinch your nose closed again, taking a moment to hold your breath.
7. Now allow your left nostril to open and start exhaling your breath, making sure that you take a moment before you began your next inhale.
8. Try to repeat this cycle of inhaling and exhaling through both of your nostrils up to a total of 10 times. Each of these cycles should take you roughly 40 seconds to complete, so the entire exercise should take you approximately 7 minutes total to do.

- **Practice Guided Meditation**

Some people believe that practicing guided meditation is one of the best ways to alleviate any type of stress or anxiety because it interrupts the patterns of thinking that have perpetuated the stress and anxiety you are feeling.

To practice guided meditation, you should sit or lie down in a place that is cool, dark, and comfortable for you. Be sure that this is a place that allows you to relax, as being relaxed is an important part of this breathing method. Now listen to some calm recordings while you focus on relaxing your body and keeping your breath as steady as you possibly can.

The guided meditation recordings will help lead you through all of the different steps that you will need to go through, but you can expect to visualize a calm, stress-free reality when you do this method of breathwork. On top of that, this style of breathing is also going to help you gain control over any kind of intrusive thoughts that you may have, which can potentially trigger your anxiety or stress.

To sum it all up, if you follow the techniques and methods that have been mentioned above, you will be able to face stressful situations without getting worked up. This will happen as you now know exactly what you can do to use your breathing to not only calm yourself down but to overcome similar situations since they will no longer stress you out. Essentially, if you do start to experience any type of stress, anxiety, or panic attack, you can now use these breathing techniques to help calm yourself and alleviate your symptoms.

If you do notice that your stress and anxiety are getting worse, be sure to make an appointment with your doctor so that you can discuss all of your symptoms and some of the possible treatments. While breathwork will help you through almost any type of stressful situation, you need to remember that your safety is always the #1 priority. This means that if you are having any type of trouble and you notice that the breathwork you do is not helping you, contact your doctor, as there may be an underlying condition that you are unaware of. Again, always make sure that your safety is priority #1.

Chapter 6: How to Use Breathwork to Calm Down

It is no big secret that a large percentage of people take breathing for granted. Breathing is just one of those things that will happen without you doing anything at all. In fact, breathing is just like blinking or swallowing; it is going to happen for you no matter what. Even when you are sleeping, these very simple acts of life are going to continue to happen, day after day for your entire life. With that being said, most people are never taught how they should be breathing, as it is simply going to happen no matter what you do.

An example that has been used before perfectly illustrates this point. A newborn baby will take some very deep belly breaths, meaning that their stomach is going to expand as much as it is able to when they inhale, and they will pull their stomach back in when they exhale that very same breath. You can use this same concept to help you calm yourself down whenever you feel as though you are starting to get worked up.

Continuing with the baby example, they breathe through their nose as opposed to their mouth, with the only exception to that being when they are congested. That said, breathing through your nose is how you are supposed to breathe. If you have paid attention to any of the breathing techniques and practices that have already been mentioned, they all have one thing in common, that being that you will need to breathe through your nose for them to work. And just as a quick reminder, every breathing practice uses the nose to inhale as it warms the air as it comes into your body and filters it as well. Your nose has been designed this way so that it can help to protect your lungs, which are very delicate.

The big question that you may be thinking is since you knew how to breathe when you were a baby, why do you breathe wrong now, after years of practice? The answer is that your modern-day life has essentially messed everything up for you. When you were a baby, you did not have a care in the world. However, when you start to grow older, you begin interacting with friends and family members, followed by school and the pressure that comes along with that. You try to fit in with your peers, as well as be liked by them. This is all going to come along with an amount of stress that is simply astronomical, and this is also going to, unfortunately, affect how you breathe as well. This is because your breathing is going to be directly related to the amount of tension that you are carrying within your body. When your body is under tension, you will start breathing in a more shallow fashion and at a rapid pace, which will occur mainly in your upper chest. When you are relaxed, however, you will be able to breathe in a fuller and deeper way, with your breaths coming from your abdomen.

If you are thinking that you can simply start breathing through your abdomen when you are feeling tense, you may be surprised to find that it is going to be very difficult to do this, as these are two different things that simply can't be done at the same time.

66

Your breath is not only the way you get oxygen into your body, but it also enhances the health of your heart, your brain function, and even your lungs. The breath that you take keeps your body cells healthy and your body operating at its maximal efficiency. Breath and oxygen unite both your mind and your emotions. Because of this, it only makes sense that you should spend a few minutes every day to try to improve this connection. And on top of that, when you can harness the power of your breath, you will be giving yourself the tools that you need to calm yourself in any situation, no matter how crazy it may be.

Here is how you can use the power of your breath to help calm yourself in any situation, no matter how infuriating it may be.

How Breathing Will Help Calm You Down

When it comes to breathwork and its ability to calm you down during a stressful situation, the number of benefits is simply going to be mind-blowing. With that being said, here are some of the ways that breathwork is able to help calm you down and what you can expect when you utilize it in a stressful situation.

- Your brain requires a lot of oxygen, more than any other organ in your entire body. Breathing properly will not only improve your concentration but will also give you greater clarity of thought and increase your ability to deal with the situation that is causing you to get worked up. Essentially, you will be able to stay calm in situations that would normally have you worked up.

- Breathwork will help you stay calm by bringing you an emotional control and balance that most people normally don't know. With breathwork, you will be able to calm yourself as you are going to be able to better control your emotions.
- Breathwork can help you find a balance between both sides of your brain, meaning that it will be better equipped to deal with all the different aspects of your life. When you can control your breathing, you will be able to calm yourself and control your emotions. This means that you will be better balanced to get your mind right, as well as to manage your emotions. As soon as you can do this, you will be able to help calm yourself down in any situation.
- Your breathwork is going to help you improve your mental focus, which means that you will now be able to free yourself from any negative thoughts that you may have when your mind is able to wander. Since negative thoughts can really get you worked up, when you are able to use breathing techniques to calm yourself, you are going to be saving yourself from a lot of unnecessary stress.
- Another way to eliminate stress is going to be to feel connected with your mind and body. When you feel stress and anxiety, your head is going to feel as though it is spinning non-stop. When you are able to practice breathwork, it is able to help you become grounded after only a few minutes.
- When you practice breathing techniques to reduce your stress and calm you down, you are going to be excreting some of your body toxins. Many of these toxins are going to be secreted through your lungs.

- You can expect your concentration to be improved. This means that if your mind is racing, it will be much easier for you to slow it down and focus on the task at hand. This is exactly what abdominal breathing can do for you.

Whenever you are in any type of situation that you consider to be stressful, there are only two paths that you can take. You can either become overwhelmed by the situation and increase the amount of stress that you feel, or you can take a second to practice certain breathing techniques and grab that situation by the horns, meaning that you are not going to be stressed out by it and you are going to take control. No matter what you decide to do in the situation, it is going to be the breathwork that you are practicing that will help you take that situation and make it a non-factor.

Now that you are familiar with how breathing can calm you down in even the most stressful of situations, here are some of the breathwork techniques that you can utilize in order to not only calm yourself but relax at the very same time.

Shallow Chest-level Breathing to Calm Down

Many people suffer from phobias. These can include simple fear, panic attacks, and anxiety disorders. If this is something that you are suffering from, you can easily handle it by checking your breathing. If you are breathing too high in your chest, it is going to be a big problem. When you breathe in at a rapid pace, it will lead you to start hyperventilating. Once this happens, it will have the potential to cause some very serious damage, including possibly having a panic attack.

If you notice that you are breathing in a shallow manner, you have nothing to worry about. While it can possibly get you worked up, by simply taking some deeper breaths, you are going to be able to calm yourself down and destress, no matter the situation you are in. Essentially, you are going to shift your breath down to your abdomen, which is where it should be going anyway. When you do this, you are going to boost your lung capacity, which is only going to increase how efficiently you breathe.

Abdominal Breathing to Calm Down

When you need to calm yourself down, breathing is going to be one of the best ways for you to do just that and calm down. The breathing techniques that are mentioned later come from the ancient art of Yoga and can be done just about anywhere that you go. This means that you can utilize these calming techniques in the office before an important meeting, before you take a big exam, give a presentation, or even after a day that was just more stressful than normal.

When it comes to breathwork, it is divided into three different phases. Those phases are going to be inhalation, retention, and finally, exhalation. Breathwork is going to require you to focus on being able to concentrate on each individual breath that you take.

Practicing abdominal breathing to help calm you down is a very effective technique that you can use in any situation. It has already been mentioned and explained in the previous chapter, but just in case you have forgotten what the abdominal breathing process was, here is a quick refresher. There are several steps that you should take, which will include:

1. Finding a chair that allows you to sit with your back straight. Put one hand on your stomach just beneath your rib cage. Make a note of how much tension that you are feeling.
2. Starting to slowly inhale entirely through your nose. The whole idea here is to fill your lungs up from the very 'bottom.' If you are using your abdomen to breathe, you will notice that your hand on your abdomen is going to rise and fall with each breath. You do not want your chest to move very much as you are focusing your breathing into your stomach.
3. After you have taken a complete breath, take a moment and pause, following that pause with a very slow exhale. Try to keep your mouth closed throughout this entire process. You should make sure that you exhale all of the air that is in your lungs, taking a second to allow your body to let go and have a second to relax.
4. Repeating this entire process 10 times, trying to keep your breathing as smooth as you possibly can. This means that you should be inhaling and exhaling in a natural manner. Just remember that you should pause for a second at the end of each inhale and exhale. Try to count to ten with every breath; the rhythm that you follow should look like this:

A slow inhale, followed by a pause, then a slow exhale (consider this to be a count of 'one'). Follow this with a slow inhale, followed by a pause, then a slow exhale (which is considered as a count of 'two').

You can extend this particular exercise by doing a couple of 'sets' of this style of abdominal breathing. Just be sure that you remember to count to ten for each set (each exhalation is only going to count as one number). After 5 complete minutes of doing this type of abdominal breathing, you will notice a pronounced reduction in your stress and anxiety.

The Calming Breath Exercise

This is going to be one of the most effective and efficient breathing techniques that you can use to reach a deep state of relaxation very quickly. To use the calming breath exercise and reduce stress, all you need to do is:

1. Start by breathing from your abdomen, inhaling slowly as you count to five.
2. Take a pause and hold your breath for a count of five.
3. Start to exhale slowly, trying to follow a five-count ideally through your nose or mouth. Make sure that you exhale fully.
4. After you have completed the exhale, go back to your normal breathing rhythm, and take a total of two more breaths, immediately repeating steps number 1 through 3 as outlined above.
5. Continue repeating the same process for at least 3 to 5 minutes. This means you will be completing a minimum of ten cycles of five, holding for five, and

exhaling for five. Be sure that you remember to take a total of two normal breaths before you start each new cycle. If you find that you are getting lightheaded while practicing this type of breathwork, stop for half a minute and then start the whole process again.

6. During the entire exercise, you should make sure that your breathing is done in a regular flowing action, which means that you are going to be able to breathe regularly and not do any type of 'gulp' breathing.

7. For an optional benefit: Every time that you exhale your breath, try saying words such as 'relax,' 'let go,' 'calm,' or any other type of relaxing word that you can think of.

This calming breath technique is one of the most effective ways that you can calm yourself during a stressful situation. If you find that you are starting to feel anxiety or stress, start using this technique to help yourself stay calm and realize that you can handle that situation in a calm, stress-free manner.

Chapter 7: Using Breathwork to Increase Your Energy

If you are like anybody else on the planet, there have been times when you have simply felt as though an extra boost of energy could completely turn your day around. Whether that be right after waking up in the morning or during the middle of the day, you can always use a little boost of energy to help you keep going strong. When you are feeling on the tired side, you may even rely on coffee or some type of energy drink to get the boost that you are looking for. However, you can use your breathing to get that same boost, but without the side effects that caffeine and energy drinks can have on your body. The side effects from these drinks include stress on your adrenal glands and your kidneys, so why wouldn't you want to try an all-natural alternative that doesn't come along with any of the negative side effects?

If you have been feeling fatigued and tired throughout your day, your main concern with a solution is most likely going to be time. What can you honestly do to boost your energy levels on the spot while preserving your time to allow you to complete the task you are doing? The answer to that question? You guessed it, breathwork. In fact, there are a few different breathing exercises that are relatively easy for you to do to give yourself a quick energy boost and get out of that 'slump' that you are feeling trapped in. Now you must keep in mind that the amount of stress you are feeling, partnered with poor cardiovascular health, are going to be the main contributors to low energy levels. This is one of the reasons that athletes have so much energy at any given time, as they frequently work out and increase their stamina, as well as their overall heart health. On top of that, exercise is directly linked with having a lower stress level, so athletes and those people who tend to work out more frequently are also going to feel less stressed.

Here are some breathing exercises that you can easily perform, no matter where you may be, to increase your energy. And the best part about these exercises is that you only need to perform them for 10 minutes or less. Now keep in mind that not every breathing exercise is going to be for you, so try them all out and choose the one(s) that you enjoy the best and that give you the most energy. No matter what you are doing or where you are, here is how you can boost your energy and invigorate your day!

Relaxing Breath (4-7-8 Breathing)

Relaxing breath, which is also commonly referred to as 4-7-8 Breathing, is going to be perfect for you if you need a quick little burst of energy and don't have much time on your hands. Originally developed by Dr. Andrew Weil, the relaxing breath technique is going to involve inhaling for a set amount of time, holding that inhale for a certain amount of time, and then exhaling that breath for a certain amount of time. To do a relaxing breath:

1. Find a comfortable seat and sit up nice and straight.

2. Completely exhale all of your air through your mouth.
3. Now close your mouth and take a big inhale through your nose, being sure that your inhale lasts for a count of four or just about 4 seconds.
4. Hold your inhale for a count of seven, which should be about 7 seconds.
5. Finally, exhale all of your breath through your mouth, making sure your exhale lasts for an eight count, or about 8 seconds.

Pursed Lip Breathing

The pursed-lip breathing technique is not only going to effectively increase the amount of oxygen that you take in but will also be very helpful in terms of slowing down the speed of your breathing (which is going to be very important if you suffer from asthma and are having any type of asthma attack). Very similar to what the name suggests, performing pursed-lip breathing is going to involve exhaling your breath through your lips while they are pursed. This helps to promote deep breathing.

To correctly perform pursed-lip breathing:

1. This can be done in any position, including sitting or standing.
2. Take a deep inhale through your nose.
3. Purse your lips together and start to exhale through your mouth only (if you need a visual, pretend that you are trying to blow out candles on your birthday cake).
4. Repeat this process for up to 10 minutes.

Laughter Yoga (Hasya Yoga)

You may be wondering why laughter is on the list of breathing exercises that can help increase your energy, but you may be surprised to find out that laughter is going to be one of the very best forms of breathing exercise that you can be doing. Laughter Yoga often referred to as Hasya Yoga, involves prolonged voluntary laughter, the main goal being to stimulate and take advantage of the benefits that spontaneous laughter brings you.

A study that was done on laughter Yoga showed that this breathing exercise can improve your mood, as well as your heart rate variability. Here is one of the ways that you can very easily perform this breathing technique and get yourself a nice little boost in your mood and your energy.

1. To get started, you should warm up by standing still, using your hands to gently push down on your stomach, essentially helping you push out all of your air and say, 'ho-ho.'
2. Once you have completed this, push your hands out in front of your chest while saying 'ha-ha.'
3. Start to slowly increase the speed that you are repeating this process until you have some type of rhythmic chant going. If you would like, you can always substitute the arm movements with clapping instead.
4. Once you have a rhythmic chant going on, raise both of your arms over your head.
5. Take a big inhale and hold it for 3 to 5 seconds.
6. Now bend at your waist, allowing your arms to completely relax.

7. Begin exhaling your breath and laughing, or if you are unable to laugh, say 'ha-ha' to help yourself induce laughing.
8. Repeat this entire procedure for a minimum of 5 minutes, but no longer than ten minutes.

Humming Bee Breath (Bhramari Pranayama)

The humming bee breath is more traditionally one of the breathing techniques practiced by Yogis, but it is often called Bhramari Pranayama as well. Some of the benefits of using the humming bee breath include increased concentration, improved memory, and even a release of both anxiety and tension. This contributes to an increase in your energy.

To properly do the humming bee breath, you will:

1. Find a comfortable and sit with your back nice and straight.
2. Close your eyes and feel your face relax.
3. Take a slow inhale using just your nose.
4. Once you are finished inhaling, follow that with a slow exhale, making sure that you do so while humming (pretend that you are a bee and are humming the letter M).
5. Continue to make this humming sound until you take your next inhale, which is going to only be through your nose.
6. You should repeat this entire cycle for the next several minutes.

Breath Counting

Breath counting is a particular form of meditation that involves using a count system for each breath that you take. The whole point of using a count system is to help improve your concentration and to settle your mind more easily. Unlike some of the other breathing exercises previously mentioned, breath counting is not going to require you to inhale, exhale, or even hold your breath for any specific amount of time or in any specific position.

To practice mouth breathing, be sure that you:

1. Get into any position that you consider to be comfortable, which includes sitting, standing, or even laying down.
2. Take an inhale through either your mouth or nose.
3. Next, exhale your breath, saying 'one' (or you can also do this quietly if you are in a place with other people around you).
4. With each continuing exhale, you want to continue counting, being sure that you do not go any higher than five.
5. After the fifth exhale, start your count over from one again.
6. Repeat this process of counting your exhales up to five and then starting over at one for up to 10 minutes.

Diaphragmatic Breathing

Also referred to as abdominal or deep breathing, diaphragmatic breathing involves contracting your diaphragm, which, as mentioned earlier, is the dome-shaped muscle that rests at the base of your lungs. This is a very common technique and possibly the most used breathing technique when it comes to breathing exercises. Aside from helping to give you a nice little boost in your energy levels, this breathing technique is also going to help you to strengthen your diaphragm, which means that you will not need as much energy to breathe.

Diaphragmatic breathing was already previously covered with step-by-step instructions. If you need a refresher on this particular style of breathing, simply find it in the previous chapters.

Skull Shining Breath (Kapalbhati Pranayama)

If you are looking for one of the best breathing techniques that will give you a quick burst of energy, you may want to consider using skull shining breath and see how you feel afterward. Also referred to as Kapalbhati Pranayama, this breathing exercise will help you improve your circulation, essentially leading your entire body to become energized and feel better. As with some of the other breathing techniques that have been mentioned, this method is also going to help you to increase your concentration and alleviate some of your stress.

To do skull shining breath, you should:

1. Sit with your back straight in a comfortable chair or seat.
2. Place both of your hands onto your stomach.
3. Now take several different deep breaths, making sure that you always inhale through your nose and exhale out of your mouth.

4. Very quickly and forcefully exhale all of the air in your lungs, focusing on bringing your belly button into your spine.
5. Once all of your breath has been exhaled, take in a regular breath, being sure that you allow your stomach to expand in a natural manner.
6. Repeat this process for the next five to ten minutes.

Conquer Breath (Victorious Breath)

Conquer breath, which is also referred to as Victorious Breath, is a special breathing technique that will help you to regulate your blood pressure, as well as boost your energy levels at the very same time. It does this by increasing the amount of oxygen that is circulating throughout your body. Now keep in mind that this particular exercise may be a little tricky if you are new to breathwork and breathing techniques because it requires you to contract your throat to control your airflow.

To correctly perform a conquer breath, you will:

1. Find a comfortable chair or seat to sit on, making sure that you are upright with your shoulders relaxed.
2. Now close your eyes. Start inhaling through your nose, simultaneously contracting the back part of your throat. If done correctly, you will notice that it makes a soft snoring type of sound.
3. Slowly begin exhaling through only your nose, making sure that you continue to keep your throat contracted through the entire exhale process.
4. Repeat these steps for up to several minutes.

Three-Part Breath

Three-part breath is going to be one of the best breathing techniques that you can try to boost your energy if you are new to breathwork or are not yet aware of the many ways your breathing is able to move your body. Essentially, if you are a beginner to breathwork, the three-part breath technique is going to be a great one to try for your first time. With it, you will focus on your diaphragm at first, moving your focus to your abdomen next, finishing it up by focusing on your chest. Three-part breath is a great way to boost the amount of oxygen that is in your blood, as well as how much oxygen is circulating throughout your body.

To get started with the three-part breath, you should:

1. Find a comfortable seat to sit up straight in.
2. Be sure that your shoulders are relaxed.
3. Place one of your hands onto your belly button and start taking a deep inhale. Focus on feeling your hand rise as your stomach inflates.
4. Exhale your breath and pay attention to your stomach deflating.
5. Repeat this same process a total of five times.
6. After your fifth breath, move the hand that was on your stomach slightly higher so that it is just below your rib cage.
7. Take a deep inhale, making a note of how your rib cage is expanding, followed by an exhale where you will note how it deflates.
8. Repeat this new process a total of five times.
9. After the fifth inhale and exhale, place the hand that was on your rib cage onto your chest (you

want it to be situated right at your collarbone) and take a deep inhale, feeling your hand rise.
10. Exhale your breath and feel how your collarbone begins to lower.
11. Repeat this final part a total of five times.

When it comes to breathing to get more energy, there are many different techniques that you can use to get the results that you are looking for. All of the different aforementioned breathing techniques have all been proven to help improve your blood pressure, increase how your concentration, decrease your stress and anxiety, increase your oxygen levels and your energy levels, and much, much more.

As mentioned at the very beginning of this chapter, not all of the breathing techniques that have been outlined above are going to be right for you. With that being said, do your best to try them all out at least one time, which will allow you to then go back and decide which breathwork exercises you like doing the best (at least when you need a quick energy boost anyways). This will allow you to not only be comfortable and excited to do these breathing exercises whenever you need an energy boost, but it will also prevent the boredom that can set in if you are doing the same breathing exercise over and over.

Chapter 8: The Top

Superventilation Techniques

Close your eyes for one second and take a deep breath. Focus all of your thought on feeling the way the wave of nitrogen, carbon dioxide, and oxygen are pressing against all of the ribs in your rib cage as your lungs expand and swell. Now repeat this process.

Before you ever started using breathwork to boost your health and well-being, there is a very good chance that you actually never thought about any aspect of breathing at all, ever. This is because your body's respiratory system is unique for your body, as you are basically not only the driver, but you are also going to be the passenger as well. You can either leave everything up to your body's autonomic nervous system, which is going to be responsible for all of the unconscious actions of your body (including processes like digestion and heartbeat), or you can decide that you are going to take control of your body by utilizing the power of your breath.

To many people who practice breathwork, this is going to offer them a path into their physiology and their subconscious mind. This is where superventilation, also referred to as controlled breathing, is going to come into play. Here is what you need to know about superventilation and how it can affect your body physically.

What is Superventilation?

As mentioned earlier, superventilation is also going to be referred to as controlled breathing. While there are no scientific studies to prove it, those who practice it swear that it makes them temporarily superhuman. In fact, it is going to be this type of controlled breathing that is actually responsible for many other types of breathing techniques, some of those including the Lamaze technique, the 'just take a deep breath' technique, and even the Pranayamic breathing that is very popular in the Yoga world. Essentially, when you practice superventilation breathing, you are going to be able to expect a better melding of your body and mind, meaning that your subconscious activities and your self-control are going to be much more in sync. Again, this has not necessarily been proven by science, but there are many people who will give testament to just how powerful superventilation breathing can be.

One of these such people is Wim Hof, a Dutch daredevil who has earned himself the nickname 'The Iceman.' Wim Hof is the main leader of the people who swear that superventilation is a real thing and can help you accomplish just about any feat that you want to.

Wim Hof earned his claim to fame by running several different marathons while topless and in. The amazing part of this was that the marathons took place above the Arctic Circle. On top of that, he has also dived under ice in the North Pole and has even languished in many different ice baths for over 90 minutes at a time. He credits superventilation for all of this and says that this breathing practice has allowed him to accomplish these feats.

Essentially, superventilation is a performance-based method of breathing that is going to very rigidly regulate how your body is oxygenated. If you can use superventilation the way it should be used, you can basically expect a massive release of adrenaline to occur within your body. Along with this massive influx of adrenaline, your sympathetic nervous system response will then go into its fight or flight response. This essentially will create a very heightened sense of alertness, get you fired up to the point that you feel as though you can do any physical feat that you are confronted with, greatly increase your energy, and even boost your mood.

With all of these benefits that superventilation can bring you, you may be wondering why you haven't heard of it before or even why you are not already doing it. You need to make sure that you are practicing superventilation correctly if it is something that you decide that you are going to want to do. With that being said, here is how you can correctly perform superventilation in order to take advantage of all the different benefits that it can provide you with.

Superventilation: The Technique to Become Superhuman

When it comes to practicing superventilation, there are two different methods that you can practice. While they are going to be somewhat similar, they are also going to be completely different at the very same time. No matter what superventilation technique you decide to use though, the practice and the temp are going to pretty much be the same.

For both superventilation techniques, you should either make sure that you are sitting upright in a comfortable chair or finding a comfortable place that allows you to lay supine. This will give you the best access to creating a straight spine (you must make sure that your spine is as straight as possible for this technique to be effective), as well as allow your lungs to expand to their fullest capacity possible.

You should use a 1:1 tempo. What this means is that your breathing pace is going to be very fast, as you will need to be taking 1-2 breaths every second. To really get the full effect of this particular breathing practice, you are going to want to make sure that you are utilizing your diaphragm (which has been discussed in the previous chapters of this eBook), as opposed to the accessory breathing muscles that you are more than likely accustomed to using. If you are just starting out with superventilation, there is a very good chance that you may feel dizzy or lightheaded but know that these feelings are going to be extremely common for this type of breathing and will occur because of the changes that will be happening with the blood gasses that are inside your body.

Here is the first superventilation method and how you can start incorporating it into your regular breathwork routine:

Superventilation Technique #1: Nasal Inhale with a Mouth Exhale

- Take a deep inhale through your nose
- Relax as you exhale through your mouth

- Repeat this for 30-50 breaths in a row

If you notice that you are starting to use your chest for breathing as opposed to your stomach, take a second to slow the speed of your breathing and return your focus to your stomach breathing using your diaphragm. Once you have completed the 50 breaths, take a very deep inhale and exhale, making sure that you hold the exhale in a relaxed state until you are no longer to hold that breath. If possible, your goal here should be to hold that breath for up to 90 seconds, but that is going to vary depending on how long you have been practicing breathwork, the style of breathwork that you have been using, and even how physically fit you are. As soon as you reach the end of that breath, exhale that breath and then take another quick breath in and then hold that breath for 10 seconds. Once you have completed this version, you can now immediately move on to version 2 of this superventilation breathing method.

Superventilation Technique #2: Mouth Inhale with Mouth Exhale

- Start by taking a deep inhale through your mouth
- Relax while you exhale that breath through your mouth
- Repeat this process for 30-50 breaths total

Once you have successfully completed 50 breaths in this manner, take a deep inhale immediately followed by a big exhale, making sure that you hold the exhale for as long as you possibly can, only taking your next breath after you are no longer able to hold the exhale. Try to hold this state of exhale for up to 90 seconds if you can, but as with superventilation technique #1, this is going to depend on the factors that have already been mentioned. As soon as you are no longer able to hold your exhale, take a quick inhale and then hold that for 10 seconds. Repeat this process 3 to 5 times in total.

When you are properly able to utilize the superventilation technique of breathwork, you are essentially going to be putting yourself into a superhuman state. Again, this has not been proven with any studies, however, those who do practice this style of breathing are going to verify that these claims of feeling superhuman and being able to do superhuman feats is a real thing. This allows you to push your body to accomplish feats that you would have never thought you would be able to accomplish on even your best day. And all of these changes are going to be due to the physiological changes that superventilation has caused in your body.

How Does Superventilation Actually Work?

If you can properly use superventilation as outlined in the two aforementioned techniques, you will essentially increase the amount of oxygen in your blood, meaning that you will also have more oxygen in all of your body tissues as well. On top of that, you will have an influx of adrenaline that will take over your body, essentially giving you all of the strength that you more than likely didn't even know that you had.

To put it as simply as possible, you are packing your body full of oxygen so that it will get into all of the tissues and cells of your body. Since all of your oxygen will be going into your body tissues and cells, your brain will not be getting as much as it should. Because it will be alerted of an oxygen shortage, it will trigger your body to start releasing adrenaline so that it will flood your body. Normally, adrenaline is reserved for survival (you know, your fight or flight mechanism), however this time, you will control your adrenaline boost. Once your body receives this influx of adrenaline, you are essentially going to be able to do anything. It is kind of like when you hear about how a mom was able to lift a car up to free her child. This is because their body system had an influx of adrenaline. It is pretty much the very same thing, however this time, you will control it.

If you are any part of skeptical about superventilation breathing, you are not alone. However, there will be many other breathing techniques (some that have already been mentioned) that are able to provide you with physical effects as well. The main difference between these particular techniques and superventilation is that the other techniques are typically going to be for the short-term only.

For example, you have more than likely heard of the Valsalva maneuver. The Valsalva maneuver is when you exhale while keeping your throat closed, which in turn is going to lower your blood pressure very quickly, as well as raise your pulse. This maneuver is going to be mainly used in order to stabilize those who are suffering from any type of heart arrhythmias.

Another example is going to be the Lamaze method of breathing, which is being used by many women who are giving birth. This is because this style of breathing has been proven to help increase your pain tolerance when it is being used, as well as to help increase your relaxation. With both of these examples, some have claimed they have started to hallucinate and even feel an overwhelming sense of euphoria after practicing them.

While we currently don't understand why hyperventilation works the way it does, it is only a matter of time before it will be fully understood. The one thing that you are not able to argue with is the fact that when you do practice superventilation as your form of breathwork, you will experience some results that are simply inexplicable. With that being said, it goes to show that your body is an amazing machine that we know practically nothing about. It is going to be exciting to see where superventilation breathing can take the human race moving forwards.

Chapter 9: Breathing Techniques to Enhance Your Workouts (Before and During Workout)

Since you will be breathing roughly 20,000 times per day, every single day without fail, the way that you breathe can have a rather large impact on how you perform during your workout. In fact, if you have worked out before, you already know that as soon as your body is under any type of physical stress (the workout you are doing), you are going to start sucking in much more air since you will be breathing harder and faster. This happens because your body needs more oxygen to maintain itself. So, the fact that your breathing is going to have a significant effect on your quality of workout should come as no surprise to you.

Knowing this, you may be wondering if there is any type of breathing technique you can use before you get started with your workout to help enhance the workout you are about to do. To answer that question in one word, yes! There are specific breathing techniques that you can use before your workout to help you maximize the exercises you are about to do.

However, there are also going to be some breathing mistakes that you are going to want to avoid during your workout as well. So, before you can fully understand the different breathing exercises that you can do to enhance your workouts, you must first know what breathing mistakes to avoid. Here are the breathing mistakes that you should try to avoid at all costs whenever you are getting ready for your workout (pre-workout) or are in the middle of your workout.

Breathing Mistakes to Avoid While You Workout

When you are focused on your workout or getting ready for your workout, it is going to be extremely easy for you to forget about how you are breathing. In fact, since you probably don't really pay any attention to how you breathe throughout the rest of the day, why would you start paying attention to it before your workout? As long as you are breathing, you should be fine, right?

Unfortunately, the answer is going to be no. While nothing bad is going to happen to you by not focusing on your breathing, you are going to be cheating yourself out of better fitness and quicker weight loss results. With that being said, here are some of the top breathing mistakes that people make all the time when they are working out or getting ready to workout.

- Using Chest Breathing

As mentioned previously, chest breathing is going to be when you are breathing with the use of your breathing accessory muscles, meaning that you are using your chest to breathe instead of your diaphragm. This is because when you use chest breathing while working out, you are restricting how much air (which also means how much oxygen) you are taking into your lungs. When you breathe with your diaphragm, however, it is going to contract itself and move downwards. This is going to allow your chest to expand even more, meaning that your lungs will be able to expand more as well. The more your lungs expand, the greater the amount of air and oxygen your body will be able to take in.

But it doesn't stop there. There will also be a similar effect when you exhale and release carbon dioxide out of your body. When you exhale, your diaphragm is going to relax and move back into your chest cavity. Your intercostal muscles are going to be able to relax more, effectively causing your chest to be able to shrink more. This is going to force out more carbon dioxide out of your body.

Finally, when you use your chest for breathing, you are going to have a weak diaphragm. When you have a weak diaphragm, you are going to be much more easily fatigued when you are working out. What this means is that you will not be able to supply your muscles with the optimal amount of oxygenated blood flow that they need to maximize your workouts.

- Using Shallow Breathing

When you shallow breathe, it is going to put even more stress on your body as you are not going to get the amount of oxygen that your body needs. Instead of taking full, deep breaths, you are naturally going to start taking faster shallow ones, essentially forcing your body to start working overtime to get the same amount of air. Essentially, it is going to be more work for your body to get the same amount of oxygen that you would if you were to take slower, deeper breaths.

Why not just start breathing deeper while working out, you ask? Depending upon your fitness level, you may be more prone to shallow breathing than you think. For example, if you have poor posture (which can be from slumping over a computer all day or only working out your chest and not your back muscles), you are going to start to lose your ability to expand your diaphragm and take in those full, deep breaths that can help you increase the performance and efficiency of your workout.

- Having a Lack of Rhythm

This does not mean that you can't get out there on the dance floor without embarrassing yourself, but rather that you are unable to get into a smooth, rhythmic type of breathing. This means that it will be much harder for you to get into 'the zone' for your workouts. You have probably tried to work out when you just weren't able to get into it and know how potentially bad that means your workout can really be.

- Holding Your Breath

Whenever you hold your breath while working out, the amount of energy inside of your cells is going to take a plunge, meaning that you are going to feel much more fatigued from your workout than you should. You may feel as though your workout was much harder, but it was not better, but actually worse.

Now that you are aware of the different ways that you should not be breathing while you are working out, you may be wondering exactly how you should be breathing to maximize your workouts and boost your energy. Here is how you should be breathing before you start working out to help boost your focus, your endurance, and your strength.

Performance Boosting Breathing Techniques

If you are doing any type of strength or resistance training, the way that you breathe is very easily going to be able to help you improve your endurance and your overall performance. This is also going to be true for any type of sports or high-intensity interval training that you may be doing or playing as well. So, get ready to boost your energy, get laser-focused, and have the best workout that you have had in a while. Here is exactly how you should be breathing before you get started with your workout and while you are doing your workout.

- Use Deep Belly Breathing

Start by lying flat on the ground, making sure that your feet are either on a chair or against some type of wall (they should be on something that allows them to eliminate the effects of gravity). This position is going to make it much easier for you to recruit your diaphragm. If getting into this type of position is not doable for you, you can always do it by sitting in a chair or standing, but it is going to be most effective if you are able to lie down. Once you have found a comfortable position with your feet on a chair, take one of your hands and place it on your chest, with your other hand on your abdominal area.

For the next 1-2 minutes, take some deep, full breaths, trying your best to focus on your abdomen and how it is rising and falling with every single breath that you take. Upon exhaling your deep breath, you are going to want to make sure that you are spending just as much time on them as you are your inhalations (so you are basically going to be spending the same amount of time on your inhale as you do your exhale).

- Warm-Up Breathing

When you are warming up for your workout, it is going to be one of the best times for you to try to refocus your priorities on your breathing. Be sure that you take a little bit of extra time to stretch out and even foam roll all of your upper body, being sure that you get your neck, shoulders, and chest especially good. Next, go through the entire deep breathing process that has been mentioned earlier, which is going to boost your energy levels before you start your active warmup. When you spend some time focusing on your breathing right before you start exercising, you are going to reinforce the proper breathing techniques that you should be using before starting your actual workout. You will be happy to know that by just adding this couple of extra minutes to your regular warmup routine, you will be sucking less air than you normally would be, meaning that your workout is going to be much more efficient as well.

- Breathing While You're Working Out

While there are many different things that you will need to pay attention to when you are working out, when you are unable to incorporate the right breathing strategy, you may find that your workout is not as long or intense as you want it to be. While the style of breathing you use depends upon the actual workout that you are doing (lifting heavy weights is going to require a much different style of breathing than running on a treadmill or doing a spin class), you typically want to make sure that you are using belly breathing, or breathing with your diaphragm, making sure that you exhale whenever you are lifting any type of resistance. For example, if you are performing a bench press, you would inhale as you lower the barbell to your chest and then exhale as you lifted the weight back to the starting position.

If you are doing a workout that is more centered on cardio, your goal should be to get into more of a rhythm with your breathing, at a ratio of 2:2 (which means you would inhale for 2 steps or pedals, followed by an exhale for 2 steps or pedals). If that doesn't feel right, you can also increase that ratio from 2:2 to one that is a little bit longer, such as 4:4. No matter what the ratio you decide to use may be, just remember that your ultimate breathing goal is to get in sync with your running or pedaling cadence. When you can accomplish this, it can help to prevent any unnecessary pressure from being placed on your diaphragm.

When it comes to breathing in the mouth or the nose, there is not a ton of evidence pointing to one as a clear winner. Both the nose and the mouth are going to have their pros and cons when it comes to breathing during your workouts. Breathing through your mouth is going to be much easier and provide you with less resistance and quicker breaths while breathing through your nose is going to help warm the air that you inhale, making it much more friendly and readily usable (especially if you are working out in the cold).

The big takeaway on whether you should breathe through your nose or your mouth while you work out is going to be up to you. Try them both out and see which one fits your workouts better and feels right to you.

Now that you are aware of how you should be breathing before your workout to boost your energy, increase your focus, and just get into the zone so that you can dominate your workout and maximize the results that you are going to get, what about after your workout? Have you ever wondered if there are any breathing techniques that you could use to enhance your recovery? Here is what you should know about breathing and your post-workout.

Chapter 10: Breathing Techniques to Enhance Your Workouts (Post-workout)

After you have just finished a great workout, you not only feel good about yourself but at the very same time, you are also afraid that you are going to be excessively sore the very next day as well. With that being said, you have more than likely wondered if there is some way that you could skip the entire post-workout recovery process, or at the very least, help to speed it up so you can recover quicker. Since you are this far into this eBook and knowing what you have already learned about breathing, you may be wondering if there is a special breathing technique that you can use to help make speeding up the recovery process for your post-workout body faster. Here is what you need to know about using special breathwork techniques to help you speed up your body's recovery process after you have just dominated a tough workout.

How Breathing Affects Your Post-workout Recovery

After you have completed a tough workout, there is no doubt that your body is going to be in recovery mode. As far as your breathing is concerned with this, it is going to be what is known as Exercise Post Oxygen Consumption, or EPOC. EPOC is essentially the amount of oxygen that your body must consume after your workout to help bring it back to homeostasis. In fact, it is how scientists measure the intensity of a workout. During your workout, your body is going to use oxygen to help create the fuel that is required to complete your exercises. However, as soon as your workout has ended, your body is going to require even more oxygen to replenish your body cells. What all of this means is that there is a direct correlation between the intensity of your workout and how much oxygen your body is going to need to bring itself back to 'normal.' The more intense your workout, the more oxygen that your body is going to require to recover fully.

As far as EPOC is concerned, the entire concept will demonstrate how important it is for you to utilize proper breathing techniques after you have completed your workout so that your body can recover. This means that the breathing techniques you use after your workout should take full advantage of every breath. For example, if you are regularly doing shallow breathing once your workout is finished, you will be dumping a lot of the carbon dioxide that has built up in your body during your workout, but you are not necessarily going to be taking in very much oxygen. When it comes to your post-workout breathing, you want to make sure that you are taking in as much oxygen as you can to get your body back to its state of homeostasis as quickly as you can.

Maximizing Your Workouts With EPOC

EPOC is also sometimes called the 'after burn' effect. This means that the more intense your workout is, the larger the oxygen deficit your body will experience. The larger your body's oxygen deficit is the more work that your body is going to need to do to get you back to your normal balance. This action is going to require your body to expend more energy, so you are going to be burning even more calories to get your body back to normal. Essentially, the greater the amount of oxygen that you can deplete your body of during your workout, the more calories you are going to be burning while your body is trying to get back to its regular state of homeostasis. So, when you can enhance your breathing technique so that you are able to get even more oxygen into your body, you are going to be more efficiently burning extra calories and taking full advantage of your workouts.

With that being said, you may be wondering what breathing techniques are available to help you recover in the most efficient manner, essentially helping you to get the maximal results from your workouts. Here is how you can utilize breathing to maximize your workouts and get the best fat burning results that you can get.

Post-workout Breathing Techniques

As previously mentioned, when you can utilize how you breathe post-workout, you are going to be providing your body with the perfect environment to recover in the most effective way possible. During your workout, you are basically putting your body into its 'fight or flight' mode. This means that your sympathetic nervous system is going to be operating at full force, which will encourage your muscle fibers to break down.

When you incorporate the right breathing exercise after your workout, you are counteracting the stressful state that your body is put in with your workout. The best thing that you can do in this situation is to get as much oxygen into your body as you possibly can. When you do, you will help to decrease your heart rate, decrease your blood pressure, and even help to slow down your fast-paced, shallow breathing.

What makes breathing for post-workout recovery so great (other than the reasons that have been mentioned above) is that it has been proven to help your body better repair your muscles and help your body to recover more quickly after your workout. This is a key element if you are serious about making your body as strong and fit as you possibly can, and it helps you to prepare for your next workout. On top of that, it is going to ensure that you continue to move forward in terms of reaching your fitness goals, as well as helping you to prevent any injuries from occurring.

Now that you know exactly how important your post-workout breathing routine is in terms of your fitness and weight loss goals, here is exactly how you are going to want to breathe after you have completed your workout.

This technique is going to be extremely effective for your post-workout recovery, but it is also extremely simple. In fact, it will be a breathing technique that you have already read about earlier in this book. In essence, you will be doing a deep breathing technique. In case you don't remember how that particular breathing technique is done, all you need to do is:

1. Find a place that is comfortable for you to either sit down or lay down.

2. Take a few deep breaths to help calm yourself and focus on the recovery of your body after your workout.
3. Next, take one of your hands and place it on your stomach, with the other hand on your chest.
4. Now take a deep inhale, making sure that you do so only using your nose. Make sure that you can feel the hand on your stomach rise as your stomach expands with your breath. Your main goal is to keep the hand on your chest from moving very much at all.
5. As soon as you have finished your inhale, hold your breath for a count of 4 and then slowly began to exhale.
6. During your exhale, feel the hand on your stomach fall with your stomach.
7. Repeat this process for the next 5 to 10 minutes.

As you breathe after your workout to help improve the recovery process, you are not typically going to be thinking about it. However, with all of the benefits that it can provide you and your body in terms of recovering and getting your body back to its state of homeostasis, breathing is going to be an essential part of your workout. If somebody approached you and asked if you would like to supercharge your fitness and weight loss results by spending 5 to 10 minutes using a certain breathing technique, you are more than likely going to say, 'heck yes' and ask them for the details of the technique. Well, you were just told about that breathing technique and exactly how it can help you take your fitness and weight loss goals to the next level. You're welcome!

Chapter 11: Your Breathing Muscles and How to Make Them Stronger

No matter whether you are a professional athlete, somebody who enjoys playing sports on weekends, or just a person who is into staying healthy and being fit, chances are that you are normally going to focus on training your legs, heart, back, and just about any other part of your body that you can think of. With that being said, there is going to be a very good chance that you have never even thought about saying (or have even thought about it for that matter) that today is the day that you are going to start training your lungs. We simply don't consider training our lungs. However, not training your lungs has a downside here. There is a direct link between the breathing you do when you are fatigued and a reduction in your performance. Basically, if you allow your breathing muscles to remain weak and untrained, it is going to weaken your other muscles as well, no matter what exercises you are doing or which sports you may be playing. The bottom line here is that when you can train yourself to breathe better, you are going to start providing your muscles with more oxygen and better physical performance. So, the big question becomes, is it possible to train your lungs?

Training Your Lungs, is it Possible?

If you are anything like most of the people out there in the world, you probably don't think that there is going to be any real benefit when it comes to training your respiratory system's muscles. But you could not be any more wrong. While you may not be able to 'train' your lungs to breathe in more oxygen or exhale more carbon dioxide, what you can do is to improve the overall performance of the muscles involved with your respiratory system. When you can do this, you will be able to increase the amount of oxygen that you are able to breathe in at any given time, as well as increase your strength so you will be able to exhale all of the carbon dioxide that your body produces.

Here are some of the main benefits that you can expect to see when you do start training the muscles of your respiratory system:

- It will help you to increase your core strength, as you are going to be strengthening both your intercostal muscles and your diaphragm.
- As your core gets stronger, you will improve your body stability, allowing you to focus on the athletic activity or exercises you are doing.
- When your respiratory muscles are stronger, they are going to become more efficient as well. This means that with every breath you take, they will be utilizing less oxygen, essentially meaning that your muscles are going to start working better.

While you are not able to train your actual lungs, you can train all of the muscles that are involved with your respiratory system. As soon as you can do this, you will then start breathing much more efficiently. As soon as you can breathe more efficiently, you will have more energy available for your peripheral muscles. When you have this extra energy waiting to be used, your respiratory system is going to start using less oxygen.

What are Your Breathing Muscles?

As previously mentioned, you are unable to train your lungs as they do not have any type of skeletal muscles when they are on their own. Your breathing is going to be done using your respiratory muscles, which include the diaphragm, all of the muscles between your ribs (which are better known as the intercostal muscles), your abdominal muscles, and the muscles in your neck.

Your diaphragm is a dome-shaped sheet of muscle fiber. Its main goal is to separate your chest cavity from your abdomen, and it is the most important muscle in your respiratory system as it helps your breath. Without your diaphragm, you would not be able to inhale or breathe in. Your diaphragm is attached to the base of your sternum, the bottom-most parts of your rib cage, and your spine. When your diaphragm is contracting, it is going to pull itself downwards toward the bottom of your stomach, principally increasing the diameter and length of your chest cavity, thus allowing your lungs to expand. While this process is happening, your intercostal muscles are going to help to move your rib cage, thus aiding in the entire inhalation process.

When it comes to exhaling or breathing out, it is normally going to be a passive movement whenever you are not exercising. It is due to the elasticity of your chest wall and lungs, which are going to be actively stretched while you are inhaling, they will both return to their regular resting shape, meaning that the air inside your lungs will then be exhaled.

When your diaphragm contracts, you inhale. When your diaphragm relaxes, you exhale. This is precisely why when you are resting, you are not going to need to apply any type of pressure to exhale the air in your lungs. However, if you are doing any type of intense exercise, you will need several muscles in order to properly exhale. These muscles are going to include the most important muscle involved with the breathing process, your abdominal muscles. Your abdominal muscles contract, which will then raise the amount of abdominal pressure you have. This, in turn, pushes your relaxed diaphragm upwards and against your lungs. When this occurs, it forces all of the air out of your lungs.

The muscles involved with your ability to breathe are only going to be able to work correctly if the nerves that connect them to your brain are intact and working. In the case of several different types of back and neck injuries, your spinal cord may become severed, which would then break any nervous system connections that there may be between your brain and your breathing muscles. When this occurs, it is only going to be bad news as you will die unless you are set up with some type of artificial ventilation.

Making Your Breathing Muscles Stronger

By now, you should know exactly how important breathing is to maintain your overall health and wellbeing.

You have already read about the way your breath affects every single one of your vital body systems, all the way down to the most basic cellular level. On top of that, breathing is going to have the power to impact your memory, how well you sleep, the amount of energy that you have, and even how well you can concentrate. Despite of all the benefits that better breathing is able to bring you, it is understandable that you simply don't have any time in your already too busy day to spend time working on strengthening your respiratory muscles. In fact, finding time to strengthen these muscles is often much easier said than done.

Having poor posture (which can be caused by hours of hunching over a computer or even a steering wheel), suffering from excessive stress, being under a large amount of mental pressure, being unable to get much movement throughout the day, and even having some conscious and unconscious movement patterns, are all going to be contributing factors to having shallow, restricted breathing and excessive tension in your diaphragm. This is going to be very bad because, as mentioned previously, your diaphragm is going to be your main breathing muscle. While you are more than likely not going to have a clue whether you are breathing poorly throughout your day, the effects of this can potentially become very serious. On top of that, the way that you breathe (or that you don't breathe, for that matter) is also going to influence how well your muscles will work.

To strengthen your breathing muscles (mainly your diaphragm), you should focus on your core. While more often than not, your diaphragm is not going to be considered a part of your core (at least in context), but it is the muscle that is located right at the base of your abdomen muscles. This means that it connects to many of the stabilizers in your body. Being part of your intrinsic core, your diaphragm is going to have a very close working relationship with your body's pelvic floor, the deep muscles of the abdominals, and even the multifidus muscles that are in your lower back. Think of these intrinsic core muscles as a pressurized pot. In this illustration, the pelvic floor is the bottom of the pot, the back muscles, and deep abdominals are the sides of the pot, and your diaphragm is the lid on the pot. As soon as one of these muscles is unable to perform its function exactly how it should, your pot is going to start losing some of that pressure. When this happens, it means that you will start to see a weakening of your stable base that helps you to effectively move as well as breathe.

If you have an overactive diaphragm, it can also cause you to have strained breathing and create neck tension too. Your neck muscles are secondary breathing muscles, which means that they, too, are often going to be involved with issues involving your diaphragm and the rest of your core muscles. For example, have you ever felt your neck start to tighten up when you are doing some type of ab workout? This happens when you do not have adequate core strength, and your neck tries to help compensate for that.

Now that you are aware of your breathing muscles and how important they are when it comes to your breathing, it is time to start strengthening them!

Ways to Help Strengthen Your Diaphragm and Boost Your Breathing Power

You now know the importance of breathing to boost your energy, increase your focus, improve all of your body systems, and just help make you feel better overall. So it's time to start working on strengthening the muscles of the respiratory system. Here is how you can get started with strengthening your diaphragm and making your breathing muscles stronger.

There are going to be three main methods that you can use to strengthen your diaphragm and other respiratory muscles at the very same time. Keep in mind that this is going to be just like exercising any other muscle, meaning that you will need to do the exercises more than one time to see any results. Muscles just don't work that way, or everybody would be fit after their first workout. With that being said, start out by trying one of the exercises below, or all of them together. You need to remember that if you don't take action, you are not going to be able to boost your breathing muscles and make them stronger.

Here are the top three exercises to strengthen your diaphragm and boost your body's ability to breathe more easily:

Stretching Your Diaphragm

1. To get started with the stretching of your diaphragm, you should start by finding a comfortable space that allows you to lie down on your back with your knees bent and your feet flat on the floor, placed hip-width apart.

2. Now take your hands and place the heels of your palms onto your thighs, right next to where your hip creases.
3. Take a few calm breaths through your nose.
4. After taking a deep inhale and a complete exhale, think about doing another huge inhale without letting in any air. At the very same time, push your hands into your thighs. Now suck in your belly, making sure that you expand your ribs to help create a sort of vacuum that is going to pull your diaphragm upwards towards your thorax. As you continue to pull your diaphragm into your thorax area, if you want to add a little extra stretch, try to make smaller movements to help bring your pelvis and spine into flexion, lateral shifts, and extension.
5. Hold this position for as long as you can comfortably.
6. As soon as you are no longer able to hold this position, relax and slowly start to inhale fully.
7. Breathe regularly for a couple of cycles and then repeat the entire process up to 5 times in total.

Activate Your Transverse Abdominis Muscle

This exercise is going to be done in two different steps. For step 1, you should:

1. Start by lying on your back in a comfortable space, bending your knees so that your feet are hip-width apart and flat on the floor, using a 'Yoga' block (a firm pillow can be substituted if you do not have a Yoga block or something similar) that has been placed between your thighs lengthwise.

2. Making sure that your lower back and pelvis are both in a neutral position, take your fingertips and place them on the lower part of your abdomen, right between your front hip bones (also referred to as ASIS).
3. Take a few breaths to relax, the last one making sure that your belly button drops down, engaging your pelvic floor, and then began to squeeze the block that is between your thighs.
4. Now feel around for your transverse abdominis (also referred to as your TVS), as it should be popping up in the same area that your fingertips are located. On a side note, it is going to be essential that you can maintain the neutral curve in your spine as your stomach is dropping.
5. Take an inhale, softening and relaxing your belly as you do so.
6. Repeat this process 3 to 5 times to really find the deep activation of your core muscles.

Now that you have completed step 1, you can now move onto step 2. For step 2, you should:

1. At the end of the last exhale, lift both of your feet one inch off the floor. Make sure that you are keeping your pelvis stable and your belly in. Double-check to make sure that your spinal curve has stayed the same.
2. Hold this position while you take an inhale, which upon completion of the inhale, lightly place your feet back onto the floor. You want to try and keep this movement as small as you possibly can so that it allows you to feel all of the subtleties of activating your muscles.

3. Pay attention to any tension that may be present in your chest, back, shoulders, jaw, or neck areas. If you do need to modify this position, do so by starting to lift one foot at a time without using the Yoga block (or whatever you are using for this).

Practice Straw Breathing

1. Start by finding a comfortable area that allows you to lie on your back, making sure that you have some type of support for your head and upper back. You are going to want to make sure that the position you are in is very comfortable.
2. Allow for your shoulders to begin falling back, opening your chest.
3. Taking a straw and putting it between your lips, take an inhale through your nostrils and exhale it through the straw that is pursed between your lips. When you breathe out through a long straw, it is automatically going to make your exhale much longer than your inhale.
4. Allow yourself to slow your pace of breathing gradually, and after a few more breaths, you should notice that there is a natural pause that happens after you complete your exhale.
5. Use this pause to rest until your next inhalation starts spontaneously, similar to the way a ball that you are holding underwater will bounce up after it is released.
6. Focus on keeping your breathing as easy as you possibly can. Have faith that your body will start your next inhale as soon as it needs to on its own, not because of your conscious efforts.
7. Repeat this process for a minimum of 3 minutes.

Those are the three different breathing techniques that you can use to strengthen your breathing muscles, which will, in turn, will make it feel as though you have strengthened your lungs. As mentioned previously, you can do all three of these different techniques concurrently or simply do one at a time and rotate them every day. No matter what you do decide to do, just make sure that you start. It's hard to improve the strength of your breathing muscles when you are never able to get started with the proper exercises.

Chapter 12: Breathing Techniques to Improve Your Meditation

From your birth, all the way to the very last moment of your life, you are going to be breathing. You can hold your breath for a short period of time, but you are never going to be able to stop breathing completely without causing some very serious damage to your entire body and overall wellbeing. Whenever you get scared of something or do some type of intense physical activity, you are going to start breathing much faster, and whenever you feel relaxed or have fallen asleep, you are going to start breathing slower. While there is a good chance that you have never spent any time paying attention to the way your body breathes all on its own, there may be times in your life that you simply forget how to breathe altogether (but only for a couple of seconds). With that being said, there is only going to be one activity when you must pay attention to your breathing, and no, it is not going to be related to any type of swimming at all.

What is the activity that forces you to focus on how you are breathing, you ask? That would be none other than meditation of course! If you have any familiarity with the different Yoga practices that have grown to become much more mainstream over the past several years, you are more than likely already aware of the fact that proper meditation breathing techniques are going to be extremely important if you really want to get your mind and body synchronized. When you are meditating, the most important thing to focus on is how you are breathing. If you are not able to master the proper breathing techniques while you are meditating, then you are more than likely not going to be able to achieve your desired results. This is why, no matter your reason for meditating, you must make sure that you are able to learn how you should be breathing.

Meditation Breathing for Beginners

If you are looking to enjoy meditation and everything that it can bring into your life, you don't have to be any kind of Yoga Guru or special Buddha. When you do begin practicing meditation on a regular basis, it is going to be very beneficial for you and will help you feel relaxed and calm, as well as help improve your overall health. Studies have shown that when you practice a regular meditation routine, you are going to be more likely to decrease the amount of fatigue that you feel throughout your day, increase your ability to manage different types of stress that you face every day, boost your heart's health, reduce any hypertension you may be experiencing, and even improve how quickly you are able to relieve the symptoms of migraines.

Since meditation is not going to require any additional equipment or skills, you can literally do it just about anywhere that you want to, at any time that you feel like it. On top of that, you can spend as much or as little time as you wish meditating as well. Essentially, it does not matter who you are or what your circumstances may be; you can practice meditation on a regular basis.

If you are new to meditation or are thinking about giving it a try, it may be a little difficult for you to immediately find your ideal state of meditative relaxation. But fear not, here is everything that you need to know to use your breathing to improve your meditation, which is basically going to supercharge your results.

When it comes to using your breath to improve your meditation, there are going to be several things that you must make sure you do first. Only then will you be able to really maximize your breathing technique to improve your meditation.

1. **Pick a Time That Works Best for You and Start Small**

Were you aware that the Buddha would spend his time sitting under a Bodhi tree with his only intention being to remain in that one spot until he was able to achieve enlightenment? While it is not really known how long he was sitting there waiting for enlightenment to find him, it was very likely to have been weeks, all of those being without any kind of food. Good news for you, however, as you are not going to need to do anything like this at all!

When it comes to getting started with meditation and breathwork, start small. If you ask anybody who practices meditation on a regular basis (for whatever the reason may be), they are more than likely going to do so during the morning hours, usually upon just waking up. In fact, there are some people who even get up at 4:30 in the morning to practice the 'Sadna' technique of meditation, which is a pre-dawn style of meditation that is done when your 'spiritual energy' is extra strong. However, there are others who enjoy meditating later in the afternoon or the early evening after they get off work or eat dinner. No matter when you decide that you are going to spend some time meditating, be sure that you can make it work with your schedule and your lifestyle. This is going to be the only way that you will be able to make it a regular part of your day.

Practicing your deep breathing techniques right before bed is going to be a great way to help you get ready for bed, but on a side note, when you practice meditation before bed, you are more than likely going to give yourself a boost of energy instead. This is because when you meditate, there is the potential to trick your body and brain into thinking that you have already gotten enough sleep for the day. With that being said, you must be realistic about yourself and when you are actually going to be able to get your daily meditation in.

When you are just starting out with meditation, you may wonder how long you should sit there and focus on your breathing at any given time. The answer to that question is going to depend on you. For most beginners, a session of 15-20 minutes is considered a great session. At the same time, even being able to spend just five minutes on your breathing and meditation is going to be extremely beneficial. If you are unsure where you should start, start small and build it up to something bigger. For example, for your first week of breathwork and meditation, try to do five minutes per day. For your second week, bump that up to 10 minutes per day. Each week you can add five minutes until you build up to 20 or 30 minutes for each session.

2. Find Your Perfect Meditation Spot

After you have practiced meditation and breathwork for a while, you will more than likely be able to do it just about anywhere, no matter how loud it may be and how many distractions there are. With that being said, if you are just starting out with meditation, you are more than likely going to need to find a spot that you can sit and focus on your breathing without any distractions for the duration of your session. While light should not really be an issue, many find that an area with lowered lighting is going to be much more calming than an area that is fully lit. Other people will tell you that they enjoy doing their breathwork and meditation outside in the sun, maybe next to a river or some other type of natural habitat. No matter what, be sure that you can find a location that relaxes you, as this is the entire point of meditation and practicing your breathwork. With that being said, you may need to practice meditating in several different areas until you are able to find the location that best suits you.

3. Meditation Equipment

As mentioned previously, you are not going to need any type of equipment to meditate and practice your breathwork. However, at the very same time, there are going to be certain items that can help you relax and set the mood for you.

For starters, no matter if you are sitting down or lying down, you may want to have a pillow to help you get more comfortable. If you are sitting, then you can use the pillow to sit on. If you are lying down, you can use the pillow to rest your head on. You may even want to use a chair or lean against the wall if that is more comfortable for you and helps you to relax. Just keep in mind that the entire point of practicing breathwork and meditation is to be as relaxed as you can be, which means that you are going to need to be as comfortable as you can be as well.

Next, you may want to consider using incense or a scented candle, or even music to help you enhance your breathwork and meditation session. While these items are not going to do much for your breathwork, they will help you get more comfortable, which is the ultimate goal of meditation. If you do decide that music is going to be part of your session, try to listen to something that has no melody, such as bells, chimes, or random nature sounds. If you choose to use music that includes words and rhythm, you are more likely to be distracted and not completely focused on your breathing.

Finally, a kitchen timer (or even the timer on your phone) is going to be very helpful when it comes to timing your sessions. If you are just starting out with meditation and breathwork, and your goal is to do a 10-minute session, a timer is going to be the perfect way to make this happen without having to worry about the time. Simply set the timer for the amount of time you would like to meditate, and then start to focus on your breathing. As soon as your timer goes off, you know that you have completed your session.

4. Which Posture are You Going to Use?

If you are just starting out with meditation, one of the biggest problems you are going to have is deciding how you should be sitting. Body posture and different breathing techniques are interconnected but isolated at the very same time. Before you can choose the proper breathing technique, you must first choose the proper posture. If you are unable to get into a comfortable position, you can be certain that your mind is not going to be in a relaxed state, as you are more than likely going to constantly be thinking about the extremely uncomfortable position that you are in and how you hope that the entire thing is over soon. This is the reason that you will first need to figure out your posture for practicing meditation, even before you decide which breathing technique you are going to use.

Now keep in mind that there are going to be no restrictions on your pose while you are meditating, as long as you are doing it for yourself. This means that your comfort is going to need to be at an all-time high so that your relaxation level follows suit. When it comes to meditation, there are several different positions that you can try. Just be sure that whichever one you choose is one that allows you to really be relaxed and comfortable. If you are not able to figure out which posture is the best on your first try, don't worry. Take a few sessions to try all the different poses a few different times, allowing yourself to make the best decision after going through all the different postures.

Here are the different postures that you should spend some time experimenting with:

- **Sitting Meditation** – This is going to be just like it sounds. Simply sit in a seat or chair and rest both of your hands on your lap. Make sure that your feet are flat on the floor, roughly shoulder-width apart. Slowly start to inhale and exhale. If this is for you, great! If not, move on to the next posture.

- **Kneeling Meditation** – If you suffer from weak or injured knees, there is a very good chance that this posture is not going to be for you. However, at the very same time, there are many people who find this posture to be the most comfortable one of all. Start by kneeling on the floor, making sure that you sit down on your legs, which will be tucked underneath your butt. If you are doing this correctly, your shins are going to be lying flat on the floor, your calves touching the backside of your thighs. To reduce the amount of pressure that is potentially going to be on your knees, you can always use a cushion to sit on, that cushion being between the top of your lower legs and your butt. Essentially, you are going to be sitting on the cushion that is on top of your legs.

- **Standing Meditation** – If you are a beginner to meditation, standing meditation may not be the best way to get started. This is because it is going to require much more concentration than any of the other meditation postures. What this means is that you will not be able to allow your body to fully relax, which is exactly why you are getting started with meditation in the first place. To do standing meditation, all you are going to need to do is to simply stand up straight, making sure that your feet are shoulder-width apart, your toes slightly pointing outwards. Now you can get started with your breathwork, being sure that you maintain this standing position.

- **Lying Meditation** – Being one of the most effective and easiest postures of meditation, lying mediation is going to be the most effective to relax all of your muscles. It is for this reason that it is the best posture for you if you are just getting started. And yes, lying meditation is going to be just as simple as it sounds. Find a comfortable place that allows you to lie down and relax on your back. If you want, you can bend your knees so that your feet will be placed flat on the ground, if it makes you more comfortable than having your legs extended straight out.

- **Seven Point Meditation Posture** – This is going to be the most popular posture, but not for the reason that you may think. While meditation and breathwork are centered on being as comfortable as you can be, this posture has been made popular thanks to the media. Anytime that you see somebody meditating in a movie, television show, magazine, or even on the internet, there is a very high chance that they are going to be doing the seven-point meditation position. To use this posture, start by sitting with your legs in front of you and crossed. Be sure that you are keeping your back as straight as you possibly can, setting your hands onto your thighs, palms facing downwards. Another technique is to place your hands on your knees with your palms up towards the ceiling. Now relax all of your face muscles, doing your best to avoid any kind of flexing of your jaw or eyes.

Proper Breathwork to Enhance Meditation

Once you have decided which posture you are going to use, it is now time to find the perfect breathing technique for you to practice. Now keep in mind that there are going to be many different breathing practices, and you can very easily try all of them until you find one that you prefer, as you can combine several different breathing techniques into each of your meditation sessions as well. When you can practice meditation on a regular basis, it is going to help you clear your mind from all of your harmful thoughts, reduce your stress, and even improve your overall well-being. Here are some of the best breathing techniques that you can start using today to maximize your meditation routine.

Simply Breathing

This is a type of breathwork that is referred to as Shamatha and is fundamentally going to be an awareness of how you breathe. One of the more common types of meditation practices, this is often referred to as the 'reset breath,' that can bring you back to your present. Studies have shown that this particular technique helps you to increase your attention levels and decrease the possibility of getting age-related cognitive decline as well. This is going to be one of the best breathwork techniques that you can use with meditation if you are new to meditating. That is because this practice allows you to become familiar with your regular breath and your innate peaceful nature.

To do this breathing practice:

1. Start by standing or sitting, making sure that you feel the weight of your body through your feet or body.
2. Make sure that you are standing or sitting with your back as straight as possible.
3. Now soften your gaze and try to fixate on one point, either in front of you or on the ground.
4. Connect to the natural rhythm of your breathing, making sure to feel every breath as your belly rises and falls.
5. Focus on this for the duration of your meditation session.

Diaphragm Breathing (also referred to as Kundalini)

With this form of breathwork, your breathing is going to center itself around the energy that is moving throughout your body with the use of certain breathing techniques. The main breathing technique involved is going to be diaphragm breathing. As explained earlier, your diaphragm is the most important muscle when it comes to how you breathe. When you can teach your diaphragm how to breathe correctly, it will help strengthen it at the very same time. When you utilize this particular breathwork technique, you can expect your body to take in more air while decreasing the amount of oxygen that you require at the very same time.

While it has been mentioned previously as a reminder, in meditation, this is how you should practice diaphragm breathing:

1. Find a comfortable position lying on your back or sitting down, making sure that you place one of your hands on your chest and the other hand on your abdomen, ideally right on top of your belly button.
2. Take a deep breath through your nose and feel how your stomach rises with your breath. Notice how the hand on your chest is not moving, and try to keep it this way for the duration of your meditation session.
3. Focus on making deep inhales that fill your lungs completely, as opposed to shallower breaths that only fill the chest. Again, the main focus here is to make sure that you are breathing with your diaphragm and not your chest.
4. Repeat this for at least 5 to 10 minutes.

Alternate Nostril Breathing (also referred to as Nadi Shodhana and Pranayama)

Being very similar to diaphragm breathing, alternate nostril breathing is going to be a special type of meditation breathing that turns all of your focus to your body and finding that internal balance. If this sounds familiar, that is because it was explained earlier in this eBook, but as a refresher, here is what you can expect from alternate nostril breathing.

Alternate nostril breathing is a special type of breathwork where you breathe through only one nostril at a time, making sure that you are manually closing the other nostril to alternate your body's airflow. You then switch the nostrils that you breathe through and exhale through.

This type of breathing has been proven to help you reduce your blood pressure while increasing your alertness.

If you are interested in practicing alternate nostril breathing, which again, has already been explained in-depth, but for the practice of meditation, you are going to want to make sure and practice this type of breathwork as outlined below:

1. Find a spot that allows you to sit comfortably, resting your right hand on your knee.
2. Now take your left thumb and use it to close your left nostril.
3. Start inhaling slowly through your open right nostril, immediately closing it with your ring finger as soon as you have completed your inhale.
4. Take a moment to focus on your breath at this time.
5. When you feel the need to exhale, do so through only your left nostril.
6. Repeat this process with each nostril 5 to 10 times per side.

Breathing Until Your Breath is Soft (also referred to as Zhuanqi)

According to Taoist meditation techniques, the emphasis is on quieting your mind and body to find perfect harmony with nature. Breathing until your breath is soft is very similar to Buddhist meditation, as it is going to be a meditative type of breathing that aims to unite every breath you take, as well as to help your mind focus on that same breath until it has become soft. What this means is that you should pay attention to your breath until it has become quiet. This type of breathwork is going to utilize your abdominal muscles to help push out your diaphragm, meaning that you are going to be pushing all of the air out of your lungs.

To correctly do the breathing until your breath is a soft technique, you should:

1. Find a place where you can comfortably sit with your back as straight as it can be. Make sure that your eyes are half-way closed and fixated on the tip of your nose.
2. Start breathing with your abdomen until your breath becomes quiet or soft.
3. To effectively use your abdomen muscles for breathing, put your right hand on your stomach, and put your left hand on your chest.
4. Take a deep breath and pay attention to which hand is moving more and the direction it is moving in. Your ultimate goal is for the hand on your abdomen to move much more than the hand on your chest, for both the inhale and exhale motion.

Intermittent Breath Retention (also referred to as Kumbhaka Pranayamas)

Intermittent breath retention is a special breathing exercise that takes advantage of intermittent breath-holding, which normally follows an inhale or an exhale. This pause of breath is ideally going to be shorter than that of the inhale or the exhale that you make. When you can hold some air in the lungs after you inhale, it is going to be known as Antara Kumbhaka. When you momentarily hold your breath after you exhale, it is referred to as Bahya Kumbhaka.

A study has found that being able to incorporate holding your breath for even a short amount of time was associated with an increase of oxygen by 56%. On top of that, another study determined that intermittent breathing is extremely useful in preventing several different metabolism issues that arise from the changes in your body. It also is effective in utilizing and burning the oxygen that you breathe with every breath.

If you are interested in trying intermittent breathing retention, you should:

1. Find a comfortable sitting position that allows your spine to be upright.
2. Exhale all of the air in your lungs by exhaling through your mouth.
3. Shut your lips and use only your nose to inhale a deep, slow breath until you feel that your lungs are as full as they can be.
4. Hold this air in your lungs for a count of 3 to 5 seconds, slowly exhaling after the hold is over.
5. Once your lungs are completely empty, try to hold your empty lungs for 3 to 5 seconds, making sure to take an inhale after this time has elapsed.

No matter if you are someone who has been meditating for many years or if you have just started, you are going to discover some of the very best breathing techniques to boost your meditation practices to the point where they will help you improve both your short-term and long-term health benefits. There are many people who think that meditation is only going to be able to help you feel less stressed out. However, you should know by now that there is much more to it than just that. Meditation and breathwork are going to transform your entire life into one that you never even thought possible. With that being said, the only thing you have left to do is to get started!

Chapter 13: Building a Daily Breathing Practice to Meet Your Needs

If you are looking to hire your own personal breathwork coach, you must be honest with yourself and know that they are more than likely going to be very expensive. While the great ones are going to be worth their weight in gold and then some, they will be able to help you create some very amazing changes in your life in just a short amount of time. However, hiring a dedicated trainer is more than likely going to be way out of your budget. If it wasn't, you would not be reading this eBook because you would have already hired an expensive breathing coach.

However, just because a good breathing coach is going to be on the more expensive side, this does not mean that you are not going to be able to get the same benefits from a very intelligent and well-designed breathwork program! You are about to learn exactly how you can create your very own breathwork program that will help you to achieve all of your breathwork goals. Basically, you are not only going to discover how to think like a breathwork trainer, but you are also going to learn how to become a breathwork trainer. This means is that you can expect to get all of the results that you want, but without having to spend all the money on an expensive breathwork coach.

Building the Perfect Breathwork Schedule

Having made it this far into the eBook, you should already have some idea of how often you are going to start incorporating breathwork and mediation into your daily routine. There are going to be five different factors that you will need to consider when it comes to building your breathwork plan.

Here is what you need to do to create the perfect breathwork plan for your daily lifestyle:

Decide Your 'Work' Days and Your 'Rest' Days

When it comes to your breathwork schedule, consistency is going to be key. In fact, consistency is the number one thing that you can do if you want to get good results. You are going to need to train your lungs often and over a period of time on a regular basis. With that being said, the very first thing that you will need to consider is how you will create a breathwork program that will keep you involved and in the game. Now, keep in mind that even the absolute best breathing workout in the entire world is essentially useless if you don't actually do the workout. If you are not serious about improving your breathwork, you are simply not going to achieve any of your goals. If you don't want it, you are not going to achieve it. The same is going to be true in every single aspect of your life.

At the end of the day, you are going to need to build a breathwork program that is not only beginner-friendly but doable at the very same time. This means that you need the right combination of rest and activity. Combining these two things is actually not quite as easy as you would think. In essence, you are going to need to plan out a small part of your day from Monday through Sunday.

Here is how you can plan out the days that you practice your breathwork and meditation techniques:

- **Write Down Your Schedule on a Piece of Paper**

Find a piece of paper and write down all of the days of the week. Now choose the days that you have time to commit to breathwork and make a note of it on this same piece of paper. Your goal should be to practice breathwork for a minimum of five days per week. This means that you are going to have two days of rest, but at the very same time, if you wish to practice your breathwork on these days as well, then you should.

When it comes to deciding on your daily breathwork schedule, there are many more steps involved than you would think.

Step #1: No matter if you already have a schedule or you are trying to figure out what works best for you, be sure that you grab a piece of paper and select the days that you can commit to your breathwork.

Step #2: Figure out what time of day you can practice breathwork without distraction. If you are a parent, trying to do breathwork around dinner time is more than likely not going to be the best idea you have ever had. With that in mind, try to find a time that allows you some peace and quiet, but that also lets you commit on a regular basis.

Step #3: Be sure that you make a promise to yourself to do the breathwork no matter what happens in your day-to-day life. Chances are that your breathwork commitment is only going to be 20-30 minutes at most, which is practically like watching a television show on cable. You should be able to commit to a television show per day to spend on your breathing.

- **Create a Breathwork Routine to Maximize Your Results**

When it comes to creating the perfect daily breathwork routine, you should make sure that you are not following the same pattern every single day. The amount of time that you spend on your breathwork, the type of technique that you are practicing, the different methods that are available to you are all going to be extremely important when it comes to creating a daily breathing routine.

When you can commit to doing the same thing every single day, it is going to be an excellent way to prevent yourself from experiencing any bodily injury or burnout that you may experience from breathwork. When you go through the same breathwork techniques over and over, you are going to be continuously pounding the same muscles. This type of repetitive stress may potentially cause you problems down the road. However, when you can tweak your daily routine to commit to your breathwork, you essentially have a recipe for success.

For this reason, you must choose a selection of different breathwork techniques that you can repeatedly do and not have to worry about your breathwork getting stale.

- **Try to Practice a Variety of Different Breathwork Techniques**

If you really want to start and stick with a breathwork routine, you are going to need to add a wide variety of breathwork routines into your day. Start by selecting your main goal. Once you do this, you will very easily be able to use that to practice all of the different breathing techniques related to your goals.

Once you have gotten settled with your breathwork routine, it will be time to take that same routine to the next level. To do this, you must increase the intensity of your breathwork routines. Here is how you can take your breathwork to a completely new level:

- **Challenge Yourself**

To make consistent progress with your breathwork, your techniques will need to get more intense. This means that you are going to need to increase the amount of time that you spend on your daily breathwork routine. As you continuously make progress, you should up the intensity of your breathwork routines as well. When you are not continuously increasing your breathwork load, you are going to get stale and eventually end up reaching the dreaded plateau.

You should not put yourself in a position that forces you to make things much harder in a short period of time. Rather, you should challenge yourself to take the time to slowly progress so that you will be more likely to stick with it. This is going to be the worst hurdle that most trainers will need to overcome. So, when it comes to your breathwork, do your best to become comfortable with your technique before you move on to the next method.

In fact, it is going to be in your best interest to practice one breathing technique for at least six weeks before you even think about moving on to a different one. This is because six weeks will allow you to not only fully understand that particular technique but also allow you to reap all of the different benefits that it has to offer you as well. Just be sure that you listen to your body and do whatever it takes to continue your breathwork routine.

How to Build Your Daily Breathwork Routine

If you are thinking about incorporating any type of breathwork into your daily lifestyle, it means that you are more than likely looking for ways to reduce the amount of stress and anxiety that you are feeling. Here are some of the best exercises that you can use to build a regular breathwork routine.

When it comes to breathing, it is not something that you have to dedicate excessive time to every single day. In fact, it is really just about setting some time aside in order to focus on your breathing and nothing else. Here are some great ideas that will get you started on this breathwork journey:

1. Start with just 5 minutes of breathwork per day. Once you get comfortable at 5 minutes, you can start increasing the amount of time that you spend on your breathwork and meditation.

2. If 5 minutes feel as though it is too long, then start with just 2 minutes. As long as you get started, you will be on the right path.
3. Be sure that you are practicing multiple times per day. Make sure that you schedule a time to practice this or that you are utilizing conscious breathing to breathe as you should be breathing.

Now that you have successfully been able to create your very own breathwork routine and schedule, all that is left is to create the best breathwork routine for you, utilizing multiple techniques. Here is everything that you need to know about creating a perfect breathwork session with multiple techniques.

Chapter 14: Creating a Successful Breathwork Session Using Multiple Techniques

In the end, breathwork is going to be a very powerful, mind-body practice that is activated with the breath that you take. While breathwork is going to be considered a special 'ritual,' it is going to be a very energetic process that you can tap into in order to get in touch with your inner self. With all of that being said, the main goal for these tips to create a successful breathwork session is going to be open as you create it, unlike many of the other tips that you have read earlier in this eBook.

If you are really looking to create a successful breathwork session, you are going to need to make sure that you have met all of the requirements. If you don't, you can expect to live a life of disappointment, failure, and negativity. Because of the positive effects of breathwork, it has been able to grow so much over the past couple of years. It is effective and can help you achieve whatever your goals may be.

If you are thinking about addressing any symptoms that may be related to a particular health concern that you may have, often all you need to do is simply breathe. Breathwork involves specific breathing patterns to help you boost your mental, spiritual, and physical health. When you can control how you breathe in certain situations, you will then be able to better focus your mind, detach yourself from any type of connection, and it will even make it that much easier to contact your inner sense of calm and peace. If you don't do breathwork, some of the negative effects may include an elevated heart rate, blood pressure, and even a much higher stress level.

How to Create a Successful Breathwork Routine Using Multiple Breathing Techniques

When it comes to breathwork, there will be a mental and physical aspect that you will need to address. Breathwork is going to be an exciting tool that can be life-changing for you. When you can reach out and start listening to your soul, it is an accomplishment on your part. Here is how you can create a successful breathwork routine that utilizes multiple breathing techniques.

Getting Prepared

Before you even think about trying to put together a breathwork routine that incorporates multiple breathing techniques, you must first be comfortable with each of those different techniques and exercises. What this means is that you are that you must practice the individual techniques one at a time, making sure that you fully understand what you are doing. It is only after you have been able to accomplish this confidence in the particular breathwork technique that you should consider combining it with another technique.

Once you do feel comfortable with multiple breathwork techniques, how you combine them into your first session is something that you are going to want to try with a particular plan in mind. Here is how you can combine multiple breathing exercises into the same breathwork session as smoothly as possible.

No matter if you are new to breathwork or if you have been practicing it for years, whenever you combine the different techniques into one breathwork session, there are some very important things that you will need to make sure to do if you want your session to be a success.

- **Always Set an Intention for Your Session**

When you can start your breathwork session with the intention of doing multiple breathing techniques, you are going to be much more likely to accomplish that goal. Knowing that you will be combining your two or three favorite breathing exercises and having that in the front of your mind will allow you to combine the different breathing techniques much more smoothly than if you were simply 'winging it.'

At the very same time, however, you must understand that if the transition from one breathing technique to another is not as smooth as you would like it to be or if you find that there is some type of problem, that is alright. While breathwork is not very difficult to do, it can be tricky when you try to combine the different techniques together. This means that it is going to be alright if you make a couple of mistakes. Just be sure that you 'fail forward' and learn from the mistakes that you made. This way, you will be able to continue to enhance and grow your breathwork routine, being sure that you are continuously bettering yourself and your technique at the very same time.

- **Make Sure You are Focused on Your Breathing**

This may sound like a no-brainer since you are practicing breathwork, but when you are trying to incorporate multiple techniques into the same session, you may find that your mind is focused on transitioning to the next breathing technique, as opposed to focusing on your current one. So, whenever you are going to be incorporating a new technique into your current breathwork routine, be sure that you are completely focused on your breathing and not transitioning to the next breathing exercise.

Plus, when you are focused on your breathing, you will notice that you are going to transition to the next breathing exercise without any trouble at all, as long as you are comfortable with the breathing techniques that you are using.

Breathwork can bring you many great benefits. It can boost your immunity and help to reduce your feelings of anxiety and stress, helping you to process your emotions and allowing you to release negative emotions. It can increase your overall happiness and wellbeing and help you to release your negative thoughts and build your self-confidence. Breathwork is a great tool you need to have in your health and fitness arsenal.

While it can very easily become overwhelming to get started with a breathwork routine as you decide which breathing techniques you are going to use and when during the day will you schedule a time for your breathing practice, the best way for you to get started is to do just that and get started. When you don't take action to actually get started, you will not be able to reap any of the benefits and rewards that breathwork has to offer you.

For example, if you are planning to start a workout routine and you buy a new pair of workout shoes, join a gym, and even get a personal trainer, if you never use those shoes, you never go to the gym on your own, and you never do anything that your personal trainer is telling you, then you are not going to get any of the rewards of your workout routine.

In the end, if you really want to be successful with breathwork, you simply need to take action and get started. Even if you have no idea what you are doing, getting started is the best and quickest way to figure it out. And once you have started, you will be able to see how beneficial breathwork can really be for you.

www.ingramcontent.com/pod-product-compliance
Lightning Source LLC
Chambersburg PA
CBHW060236030426
42335CB00014B/1484